INTEGRAL
YOGA
HATHA

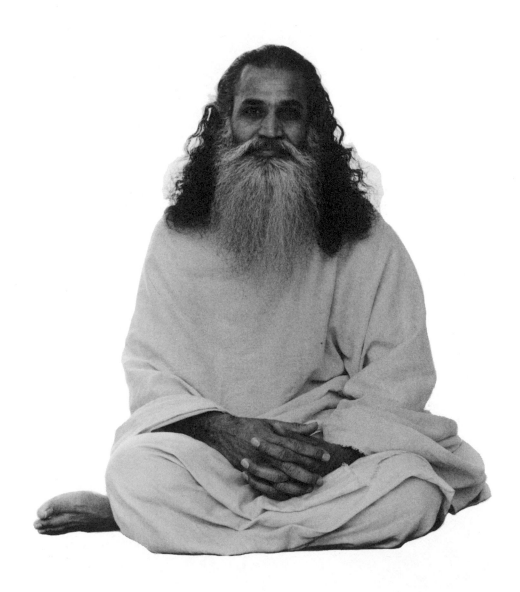

INTEGRAL YOGA HATHA

YOGIRAJ SRI SWAMI SATCHIDANANDA

An Owl Book

HOLT, RINEHART AND WINSTON

NEW YORK

Published by Holt, Rinehart and Winston,
383 Madison Avenue, New York, New York 10017.
Published simultaneously in Canada by Holt, Rinehart and Winston of Canada, Limited.

Library of Congress Catalog Card Number: 76-117272

Published November, 1970
20 19 18 17 16 15 14 13 12

Designer: Carl Weiss
ISBN: 0-03-085089-4

Printed in the United States of America

TO MY GURUDEV HIS HOLINESS SRI SWAMI SIVANANDAJI
MAHARAJ WHO INITIATED ME INTO THE HOLY
ORDER OF PARAMAHAMSA SANYAS; AND

TO ALL OTHER MASTERS FROM WHOM I HAVE DERIVED MUCH
BENEFIT IN PREPARING MYSELF IN THE VARIOUS FIELDS
OF YOGA BEFORE I ENTERED MONKHOOD; AND

TO ALL OF MY THOUSANDS OF YOGA STUDENTS ALL OVER THE
WORLD THROUGH WHOM I HAVE LEARNED EVEN MORE ABOUT
THE GREATNESS OF THE YOGIC SCIENCE; AND

TO ALL THOSE WHO WANT TO TREAD
THE GLORIOUS PATH OF YOGA.

OM SHANTHI.

CONTENTS

II

The mark over the letter a signifies long a. For example, āsana is pronounced aasana; prānāyāmās, praanaayaamaas.

"ANYONE WHO PRACTICES YOGA PROPERLY AND SINCERELY
BECOMES A SIDDHA (ACCOMPLISHED); BE
HE YOUNG, OLD OR EVEN VERY
OLD, SICKLY OR WEAK."

—*Hatha Yoga Pradheepika.*

PREFACE

WHAT IS INTEGRAL YOGA? Integral Yoga is a combination of specific methods designed to develop every aspect of the individual: physical, emotional, intellectual, and spiritual. It is a scientific system which integrates the various branches of Yoga in order to bring about a complete and harmonious development of the individual.

Every human being longs for true and lasting happiness. The path or means through which he attempts to find it varies according to the level of the individual's development. He may strive for happiness by satisfying the physical, emotional, and intellectual aspects of his personality. Experience may teach him what sages and saints have been proclaiming throughout the ages, that true and lasting happiness cannot be based on that which is impermanent in its nature. True and lasting happiness can only be attained through the knowledge of the permanent or Divine which is the Indweller of all beings and the source of all life. It has been given such names as the Self, Nature, God, Brahman, Cosmic Consciousness, Infinity, the Thing in Itself, Nirvana, and so on. Since it is infinite, it can only be experienced when the individual raises above his limited personality.

The body, emotions, and intellect must be developed to a level in which they function healthfully and in perfect harmony with each other. Only then can one live a happy life and use them as tools to transcend limitations and to experience the Divine.

SOME OF THE MAIN BRANCHES OF YOGA

Hatha Yoga: Bodily postures (āsanas), deep relaxation, breath control (prānāyāma), cleansing processes (kriyas), and mental concentration create a supple and relaxed body; increased vitality; radiant health; and help in curing physical illness. Through proper diet, the physical body undergoes a cleansing through which impurities and toxins are eliminated and at the same time vitamins and minerals are readily assimilated and utilized by the system. As the body and mind become purified and the practitioner gains mastery over his mind, he finally attains the goal of Yoga, Self Realization.

Karma Yoga: The path of action through selfless service. By performing duty without attachment or desire for the results of action, the Karma Yogi purifies his mind. When the mind and heart are purified, the Karma Yogi becomes an instrument through which the Divine Plan or Work is performed. Thereby he transcends his individuality and experiences the Divine Consciousness.

Bhakti Yoga: This is the path of love and devotion to God, a Divine Incarnation or the spiritual teacher. By constant love, thought, and service of the Divine, the individual transcends his limited personality and attains Cosmic Consciousness. The path of Bhakti or devotion can be practiced by everyone. All that is needed is faith and constant loving remembrance of God.

Raja Yoga: This is the path of meditation and control of the mind. It is based on ethical and moral perfection and control of the senses which leads to concentration and meditation by which the mind can be stilled from its thoughts. Then all limitations are transcended and the state of Samadhi or Superconsciousness is experienced.

Japa Yoga: Japa Yoga is a part of Raja Yoga. Japa means repetition of a mantra. A mantra is a sound structure of one or more syllables which represents a particular aspect of the Divine vibration. Concentrated mental repetition of the mantra produces vibrations within the individual's entire system that are in tune with the Divine Vibration.

Jnana Yoga: This is the path of wisdom. It consists of self-analysis and awareness. The Jnana Yogi gains knowledge of the Self by ceasing to identify himself with the body, mind, and ego. He completely identifies with the divinity within him and everything and realizes the oneness.

Integral Yoga is a synthesis of all Yogas. The goal is a body of perfect health and strength. Mind with all clarity, calmness, and control. Intellect as sharp as a razor, will of steel, heart full of love and mercy, a life dedicated to the common welfare and Realization of the True Self.

In this book, Hatha Yoga will be reviewed. There are many, many books on this subject on shelves and in libraries throughout the world. Because of this, I hesitated to add one more book to the market and perhaps even flood the river of existing material. It has only been through the urging of my students, who insisted on seeing my way of teaching also in print, that this book has been compiled. I truly hope it won't strain the category of Hatha information, but instead will be useful in a unique way, enabling the practitioner to gain from my personal practices and from the knowledge collected through teaching Hatha all over the globe for the past twenty-five years.

This book contains very little theoretical material, but has been set up as a sort of Hatha Yoga directory—including precise and simplified technical details plus pictures with each pose.

I now express my sincere gratitude and thanks to the students who helped me in preparing this volume, particularly to my spiritual children Sister Yoga of Ceylon and Sita and Gita of America.

SWAMI SATCHIDANANDA

New York
January 1970

A body of perfect health and strength, mind with all clarity and calmness, Intellect as sharp as a razor, Will as pliable as steel, heart full of love and compassion, Life full of dedication and Realization of the True Self is the Goal of Integral Yoga.

Attain this through asanas, pranayama, chanting of Holy Names, self discipline, selfless action, manthra Japa, Meditation, study and reflection.

Om shanthi, shanthi, shanthi,

Ever yours in Yoga,

Swami Satchidanand

ॐ

INTRODUCTION

Yoga āsanas are not exercises. The word "exercise" tends to give the idea of a practice done with quick movement and a measure of strain involved. "Āsana" simply means posture. According to Maharshi Pathanjali Bhagavan, the definition of a posture or pose means one that gives steadiness and comfort. And so, the Yoga āsanas should be practiced with the utmost ease and comfort.

Symptoms of old age, such as wrinkles and poor complexion, are caused by poor circulation of the blood, thus leaving a lot of toxins and other waste matter in various parts of the body. Once the blood circulation is enriched, however, this foreign matter is washed out and eliminated, giving the body a younger look and feel.

As the Yoga āsanas and Yogic breathing are practiced, increasing the vitality of the body, there will follow a considerable decrease in harmful acts such as smoking and drinking. Many, many Yoga practitioners have told me that, surprisingly enough to them, they had unconsciously lost the desire to smoke and drink. For that reason, I have never asked any of my students to give up habits such as the above-mentioned, nor have I used a "don't-do-this," "don't-do-that" method of training. To expect a student to get rid of his harmful habits before even starting Yoga practice would be like a doctor asking his patients to cure themselves of their ailments before receiving his treatment. Yoga is a cure-all of illness, whether mental or physical. As one takes to it, the ailments begin to disappear.

There is no better health tonic than Yoga āsanas, and, as everyone will agree, nothing is possible in this world without good health. You can have neither Bhōgā (enjoyment) nor Yoga (oneness with God) when you have Rōgā (ailment). But, when you enjoy radiant health, you can lead either a vyavahāric (worldly) life or boldly enter upon the Nivriti Mārga (renunciate path). Without good health you can expect only a cheerless existence and cannot even entertain thoughts of serving or renouncing the world.

The āsanas are effective not only in the prevention of disease but in aiding the cure of existing disease as well. From prince to peasant, child to granny, ailing to robust, all can practice these Yoga poses with the maximum advantage.

THE 72,000 NĀDIS: What are the symptoms of good health? They include —real hunger; good digestion; sound sleep; perfect functioning of the various organs of the body; proper pulsation; limited temperature; timely elimination of feces, urine, and perspiration (within proper limits); interest in doing one's duties; happiness of the mind; etc.

All these functions are properly controlled by a natural vital energy within the body, operating through the multivarious fine and subtle nerves which are spoken of by the ancient Yogis. They say there are 72,000 subtle nerves or nādis in the body, all originating in the spinal column.

The gross nervous system operates in the physical body and the subtle nervous system (nādis) in the astral body. There are subtle nādi centers in the astral body that correspond to the physical nerve centers or plexuses, and these are known as *Ādhāra Chakrās* in the Yogic terminology.

The main Chakrās are—mūlādhārā, swadishtāna, anāhata, vishuddhi, ājna, and sahasrara. The three most important nādis are the ida, the pingala, and the sushumna, which function throughout the length of the spinal cord. The sushumna functions only when the subtle, tremendous energy called Kundalini, or the "Serpent Power," is aroused and ascends through it. At this time, when the Kundalini rises through the different chakrās and reaches the highest one—the sahasrara, or "thousand-petaled lotus"—the practitioner enjoys the bliss of Samādhi.

THE ENDOCRINE GLANDS: Aside from the nerve centers, the endocrine glands also play a very important role in preserving the harmonious functioning of the body. These glands produce the very necessary secretions known as hormones, which benefit you both physiologically and psychologically. They are the pineal, pituitary, thyroid, parathyroids, thymus, adrenals, and gonads. Albert Einstein said of them, "Even our destiny is decided by the endocrine glands."

These glands are stimulated not only by your physical movements, but by your thoughts as well. An evil thought or a fit of anger disturbs your physical harmony by causing the glands to produce irregular secretions. So you should always take care of your thoughts, making sure to invite only virtuous ones into the mind.

The Yoga āsanas and prānāyāmās serve to keep these endocrine glands in perfect balance and healthy condition.

Prana is the subtle power at the basis of life. The vibration of prana causes the mind to think. When this vibration is irregular, as is usual in the normal person, thought is also haphazard. Conversely, when the vibration is regular, there is calm within.

Prana is the energy of the mind, the Commander-in-Chief of the vast army of minute cells which make up the body. When the prana is regular, the cells work in unison, resulting in harmony throughout the entire system. This all-important regulation of prana occurs through the regular practice of Yoga āsanas and prānāyāma. Thus, these along with other Yogic practices benefit us not only physically but mentally and spiritually too.

I have been asked such questions as, "We may get health through Yoga āsana practice, but what about strength?" The answer is: Through these practices you get the normal strength which everyone needs, and apart from physical strength, you get the real mental strength as well, which you need even more than bodily strength.

Those who wish to develop muscular strength and get well-formed biceps and triceps can supplement Yoga practice with other forms of exercise but should never forget that health is much more important than muscular strength. One might be able to lift heavy weights, run long distances, jump to extreme heights, break chains, swim for miles, even stop automobiles, but is he immune to illness? Even great mental ability—being able to solve involved mathematical problems—comes second to health. Having phenomenal powers of memory is of no use without a balanced mind, one that can accurately weigh pain and pleasure, praise and censure; one that is fearless, residing in permanent peace and bliss.

That person with health and strength of the physique, the mind, morality, and spirit is the real gem among mankind, and possesses the true treasure. It is my sincere wish and prayer that all of you possess such a treasure through the practice of Yoga, and enjoy supreme peace, prosperity, and Yogic bliss.

Health is your birthright, but not disease; Strength your heritage, but not weakness; Courage, but not fear; Bliss, but not sorrow; Peace, but not restlessness; Knowledge, but not ignorance.

May you attain this birthright, this Divine Heritage, to shine as fully developed Yogis, radiating joy, peace, and knowledge everywhere.

Om Shanthi. Shanthi. Shanthi!

HINTS

AGE: At all ages and in all conditions of the body—stiff, tense, flabby, etc.—you can start practicing Yoga. Those negative conditions will leave by themselves when they see you fully supple and relaxed. I have had, and am still having, students in their eighties who have just begun Yoga!

BEGINNERS: Beginners should not be in a hurry, and thereby strain themselves, to come to the perfect position at once. They should do the āsanas and other Yogic practices just to their own capacity, without the least strain. Even if the poses are not perfect in the beginning, it does not matter. Regular practice will gradually lead to perfection. The same warning applies to those who restart Yoga practice even after an interval of a few weeks.

PATIENTS: If there is any illness, it is always advisable to consult a Yoga therapist and then start the practice. This holds especially true for those who have undergone major operations or are suffering from heart trouble or abnormal blood pressure.

WOMEN: Women should suspend all Yoga practices except Savāsana (corpse pose) and Nādi Suddhi (nerve purification) during their menstrual period and also for two or three days afterward. In cases of pregnancy, if they are regular practitioners, women may continue practice for about the first three months, but they should leave out the strenuous abdominal exercises. After this, if they wish to continue practicing āsanas, it would be best to consult a Yoga therapist, as poses such as Sarvāngāsana (shoulder stand) and Matsyāsana (fish pose) may be practiced with benefit even up to the seventh or eighth month of pregnancy. After childbirth, considering the condition of the body, women can restart āsana practice after the fourth or fifth month. Those women starting practices for the very first time should not do so during pregnancy or until six months after childbirth.

CHILDREN: Sirshāsana (head stand), Mayurāsana (peacock pose), Uddhiyāna (stomach lift), Nauli Kriya (isolation and rolling of the abdominal recti), and other difficult practices are best avoided by children until the age of twelve.

PURGATIVES: Those starting Yoga practice for the first time and those restarting after a long interval would find it beneficial to take a purgative and clean their bowels before starting practice.

CONSTIPATION: Those who find it difficult to evacuate the bowels before beginning practice can drink a cup of cold or warm water early in the morning, followed by the performance of a little Uddhiyāna (stomach lift) and Nauli Kriya (isolation and rolling of the abdominal recti) or by giving the abdomen a gentle massage by hand, which will help to get the bowels evacuated.

TIME: The morning hours, when the stomach is almost empty, after evacuation of the bowels, is very conducive to the practice of Yoga āsanas. If there is a little stiffness in the body, either walk briskly for a while or perform a few Soorya Namaskārams (salutations to the sun) to remove the stiffness.

Beginners may find their bodies more flexible in the evenings than in the mornings. Āsanas may also be practiced five hours after lunch, if only a cup of liquid has been drunk during that time.

Nowadays, when everyone is busy, it may be very difficult to practice regularly in the evening. Many days' practice might have to be missed altogether due to unforeseen circumstances. Therefore, it is advisable to switch over to morning practice as soon as possible. Then, even if you happen to miss your morning practice, you can make it up in the evening.

PLACE: Yoga poses should be practiced in an airy room or in the open. Avoid hot sunshine and drafts. The ground should be level, with no uneven surfaces.

DRESS: Dress should be the bare minimum and should never be tight. No restrictive clothing should be worn. Men can wear swimming trunks or shorts. Women can wear shorts and blouses or leotards and tights.

PREPARATION OF FLOOR OR GROUND: Āsanas should be practiced on a thick rug or carpet, or on a blanket folded width-wise into four. This can be covered with a towel.

ORDER: The poses and prānāyāmās are better done in the proper order given herewith, whether done in the morning or evening. Start with āsanas, followed by Yoga Mudrās, Bandhas, and Kriyas, and finish with prānāyāmās. Kapālabhāti should be considered as part of prānāyāma.

In practicing āsanas, it is advisable that students follow the sequence of poses as given in here. While training, however, you need not follow this sequence rigorously, but pick the easiest āsanas first, followed by the more difficult ones.

TIME LIMIT: If the Yogic poses are done just for maintaining general health, adhering to the time limit as given here for each pose will bring the best results. If the practice is done for curative purposes, the time limit may vary. This should be left to the discretion of the Yoga therapist. As it is difficult to calculate the duration of each pose by looking at a timepiece every now and then, it is better to count mentally— 1, 2, 3, and so on. It would be better still if you add "OM" to your counting—OM 1, OM 2, OM 3, etc.

REST: In between āsanas, whenever necessary, one should relax in Savāsana (corpse pose). At the end of practicing all the poses, and before starting prānāyāma, Savāsana should be done for a longer time, at least a minimum of three minutes. One should see that there is no straining nor any heavy breathing at all during the practice. Even at the end of practice, one should feel quite fresh, both physically and mentally.

BREATHING: During the practice of āsanas, the breath should never be retained for a long time. It doesn't matter if you stop the breath for a moment when necessary, such as while raising the legs to form Halāsana (plow pose) or Sarvāngāsana (shoulder stand) or while raising the body to form Paschimothānāsana (forward bend). Again, during Uddhiyāna Bandha and Nauli Kriya, the external retention of the breath (keeping the breath out) comes about automatically.

As a general rule, it is good to exhale as you bend the body forward and to inhale as the body is bending backward, and to have normal breathing at all other times. It is always better to breathe through the nose and never through the mouth, except in such special cases as Sitali (cooling breath) and Sitkāri (wheezing breath), when inhalation is done through the mouth. In relieving the tension of the body while doing Savāsana (corpse pose), in the cases of the stomach and chest, exhalation is done through the mouth. Is it not better for us to remember that the nose is for breathing and the mouth is for eating and talking? If we are going to use the mouth for breathing all the time, we might as well use the nose for eating and talking!

BATHING: As a general rule, it is better to have a bath or shower before practice, but it is not a necessity. If you perspire a great deal during practice, bathing can be done about twenty minutes after the end of it. If you have not started the day with japa and meditation, you may finish āsanas with Savāsana (corpse pose), bathe after twenty minutes, and then practice prānāyāma, japa, and meditation. A cold-water bath is very beneficial, but if weather and body condition do not permit it, a lukewarm bath may be substituted. An oil bath taken once a week helps to improve health. This should be taken a little while after āsana practice, never before.

DIETETIC RESTRICTIONS: There are no "musts" about the diet, except that strong stimulants are best avoided. This comes gradually, however, of its own accord, when one practices Yoga regularly and, therefore, there is no need to worry over it. To derive the maximum benefit of Yoga practice from the very beginning, though, a pure and plain, satwic, vegetarian diet free of meat, fish and eggs is most helpful. That does not mean that a nonvegetarian diet will cause harm to the practitioner, but one cannot gain with it the same benefit that can be gained with a pure, plain vegetarian diet. Even vegetarian food becomes un-Yogic when it is fried or mixed with spices.

As for beverages, when strong drinks such as tea, coffee, cocoa, etc., themselves are not advised, it is needless to say anything further about intoxicating liquors. Again, I will stress that if one finds it difficult to change over to a Yogic diet of his own free will, it does not really matter, because, in the long run, with regular Yogic practice, cravings for unsuitable foods will slowly diminish. In the morning hours, after answering the call of nature, and ten minutes before āsana practice, it is good to drink a cup of plain water. This reduces the heat produced after the night's sleep. Those who are physically weak can drink a cup of milk.

A light snack (a piece of toast or a muffin, etc.) may be eaten half an hour after practice. A full meal may be eaten one hour after practice.

BRAHMACHARYA OR CELIBACY: The vital fluid in the body is most sacred and should be preserved at all costs. Both men and women should always remember this. It is the very life of a person. Those leading a family life should try to preserve this energy by restricting indulgence. Strict observance of continence immensely benefits everyone, and those who follow the Yogic Path will be benefited all the more.

MENTAL PURITY: The endocrine glands of the body react not only to physical activity but also to thought vibrations in the mind. For instance, if you think of something delicious to eat, you can immediately note that the salivary glands are pouring forth their juices into the mouth. A fit of anger causes the bile duct to splash bile into the blood-stream, and makes the face red. When you walk on a narrow plank bridging two high walls, the fear of falling down kindles the pituitary and makes you giddy (whereas the same act would not inspire fear if the plank were placed on the floor). Therefore, it is absolutely necessary to follow the ethical precepts of Yama and Niyama in order to keep the mind pure. Yama and Niyama form the basic rungs of the spiritual ladder and, however much you follow the physical practices of Yoga, you cannot expect to receive the higher benefits of the glorious Yogic Path unless you have mental purity.

The five precepts of Yama are: nonkilling, truthfulness, nonstealing, continence, and not accepting gifts. The five observances of Niyama are: internal and external purification, contentment, austerity, study of the Scriptures, and worship of God.

The mind must be restrained from all of its cravings, sudden fits of anger, fear, excitement, and the like. By following even one or two of the rules of Yama and Niyama, one can raise himself to lofty spiritual heights.

GAMES AND PHYSICAL EXERCISES: Unlike the rhythmic breathing in Yogic practices, breathing becomes vigorous in games and other exercises, and this vigorous breathing will disturb the particular rhythm you are trying to cultivate in the body and mind through Yoga practices. Therefore, it is always advisable not to mix up the two. Those who really wish to play games or have some physical exercises as well as Yoga practices may do so in the evenings and have the Yoga practices in the mornings. Otherwise, if both have to be practiced at the same time period, the physical exercises can be done in the beginning and, after a sufficient rest, the Yoga practices can follow.

FUN PERFORMANCE: Performing āsanas and prāṇāyāmās at all sorts of improper times, just for the sake of fun or to show off one's skill in Yoga practice, might cause serious harm.

BOOK KNOWLEDGE: Because they read in a book that Sirshāsana (head stand), Sarvāngāsana (shoulder stand) etc., if done for a long time, will bestow great benefits, many people hold these poses for a long time as soon as they become introduced to such practices. In many cases, this results in grave danger. Therefore, it is my earnest request that beginners do these poses just for the minimum time given and gradually increase the period. Even if one finds it easy to retain the poses for a long time at the beginning, it is better that one does not retain the poses for too long. Instead, the practitioner should show his enthusiasm by being regular in his daily practice, rather than by practicing for long hours some days and leaving practice completely undone on others.

PRĀNĀYĀMA: As soon as the term prāṇāyāma is mentioned, many people think that they should draw in their breath as much as possible and retain it until the eyeballs bulge and the body perspires profusely and trembles. It is, however, a great mistake to think in that way. Prāṇāyāma should be started with a simple inhalation and exhalation without retention for a few months. After that, one can start retaining the breath for a few seconds and gradually increase the period of retention to a certain limit. When that limit is reached, the number of prānāyāmās is increased, and not the duration of retention. Among the different types of prānāyāmās, Kapālabhāti (skull shining), Bastrika (bellows breathing), and Ujjayi (hissing breath) should follow, not only evacuation, but, if possible, a full bath. These are best practiced in Padmāsana (lotus pose) or Siddhāsana (accomplished pose). For Kapālabhāti and Bastrika, Padmāsana is preferable.

Prānāyāma may be practiced separately from the āsanas after Savāsana and after taking a bath. Prānāyāma will become a nice preparation before starting such advanced practices as puja (ritual worship), japa (repetition of the Lord's name, or mantra), dhārana (concentration), and dhyāna (meditation).

CHANTS

Now we are all finished with the hints to be noted for Yoga practice. Before starting practice, it is beneficial to repeat the following prayers with deep feeling and strong will. Within a short time, they will give maximum benefit. To repeat them, it is good to sit in a meditative pose.

OM   OM   OM

Om Thryambakam Yajaamahe
Sugandhim Pushti-Vardhanam
Urvaarukamiva Bandhanaan
Mruthyor Muksheeya Maamruthath.

We worship the three-eyed One who
    is fragrant and who nourishes all
    beings.
May he liberate us from death for the
    sake of Immortality,
Even as the cucumber is severed from
    its bondage of the creeper.

Om Namah Sivaaya Gurave
Satchidaananda Moorthaye
Nish Prapanjaaya Shaanthaaya
Niraalambaaya Thejase.

Om! Salutation to the Guru
who is Siva (auspiciousness),
who is the embodiment of Existence/
    Knowledge/Bliss,
who is free from world consciousness,
who is peaceful, without support and
    Self-effulgent.

O adorable Lord of mercy and love,
Salutations and prostrations unto Thee.
Thou art omnipotent, omnipresent, omniscient,
Thou art Satchidananda (Existence-Knowledge-Bliss Absolute).
Thou art the Indweller of all beings.
Grant us an understanding heart,
Equal vision, balanced mind,
Faith, devotion and wisdom.
Grant us inner spiritual strength to resist temptation
And to control the mind.
Free us from egoism, lust, anger, greed and hatred,
Fill our hearts with divine virtues.
Let us behold Thee in all these names and forms,
Let us serve Thee in all these names and forms,
Let us ever remember Thee,
Let us ever sing Thy glories,
Let Thy name be ever on our lips,
Let us abide in Thee for ever and ever.

Om Shanthi. Shanthi. Shanthi.

After finishing your practice, you can repeat the following prayer:

OM   OM   OM

Asatho Maa Sath Gamaya   Lead me from unreal to Real
Thamaso Maa Jyothir Gamaya   Lead me from darkness to Light
Mruthyor Maa Amrutham Gamaya.   Lead me from death to Immortality.

Om Shanthi. Shanthi. Shanthi.

(This may be followed by a minute of silence.)

Lokaa Samastaa Shukino Bhavanthu.   May the entire world be happy.
Jai Shree Sat Guru Maharaj Ki!

OM TAT SAT

PART ONE

NETHRA VYĀYĀMAM

or

THE EYE EXERCISES

Sit in a comfortable position, feel the body quiet down. Close the eyes and relax. In all of the following eye exercises, begin slowly, gradually increasing the speed of the movements. After ten to fifteen times, close the eyes and allow them to relax.

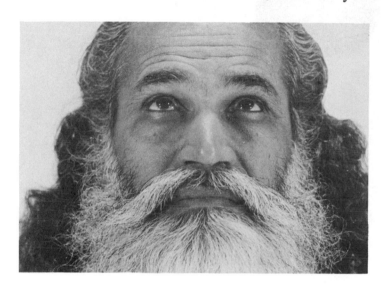

NETHRA VYĀYĀMAM—*Eyes Up*

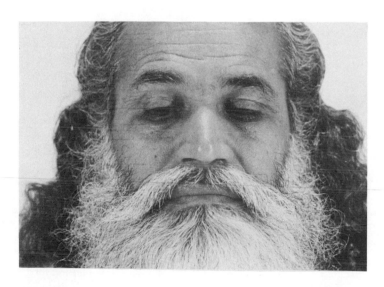

NETHRA VYĀYĀMAM—*Eyes Down*

EXERCISE 1: Move the eyes vertically, up and down, as far as they will go.

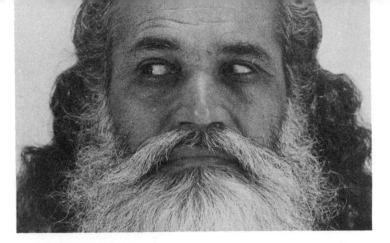

NETHRA VYĀYĀMAM—*Eyes Right*

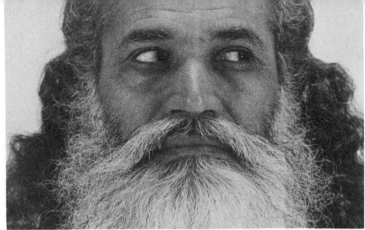

NETHRA VYĀYĀMAM—*Eyes Left*

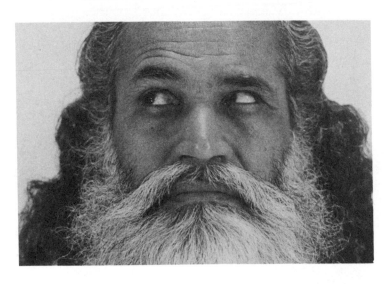

NETHRA VYĀYĀMAM—*Diagonal—Eyes Up Right*

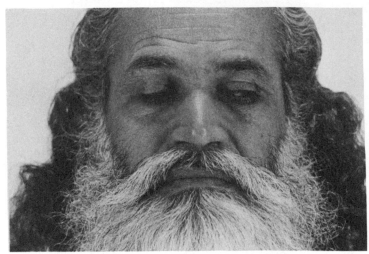

NETHRA VYĀYĀMAM—*Diagonal—Eyes Down Left*

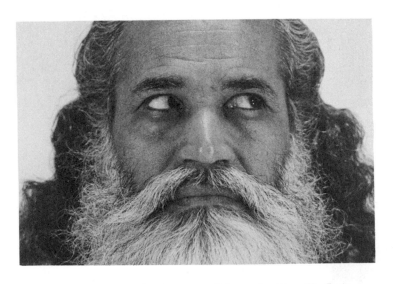

NETHRA VYĀYĀMAM—*Diagonal—Eyes Up Left*

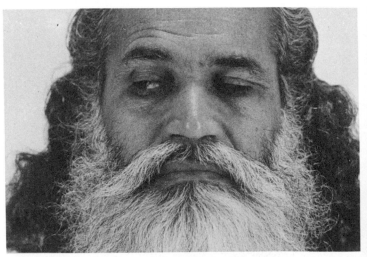

NETHRA VYĀYĀMAM—*Diagonal—Eyes Down Right*

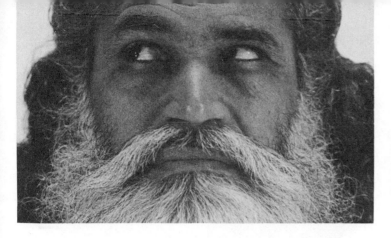

NETHRA VYĀYĀMAM—*Half-Circle—Upper Half*

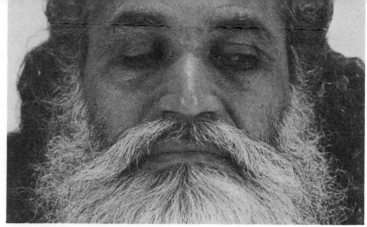

NETHRA VYĀYĀMAM—*Half-Circle—Lower Half*

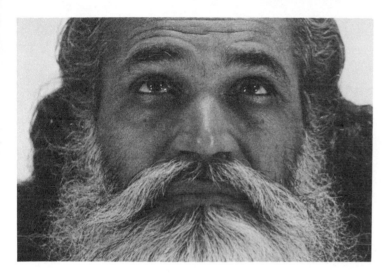

NETHRA VYĀYĀMAM—*Clockwise Circle*

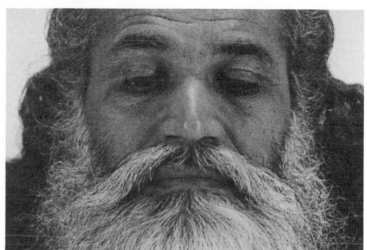

NETHRA VYĀYĀMAM—*Counterclockwise Circle*

EXERCISE 2: Move the eyes horizontally, from right to left.

EXERCISE 3: Move the eyes diagonally, from the upper right to the lower left.

EXERCISE 4: Move the eyes diagonally, from the upper left to the lower right.

EXERCISE 5: Move the eyes in a half-circle, from the lower right, up around the top half of the eye to the lower left, and back over the top of the eye to the lower right.

EXERCISE 6: Move the eyes in a half-circle, from the upper right, down around the bottom half of the eye to the upper left, and back under the bottom of the eye to the upper right.

EXERCISE 7: Move the eyes clockwise in a full circle, passing through all points on the circle.

EXERCISE 8: Move the eyes counterclockwise in a full circle.

[5]

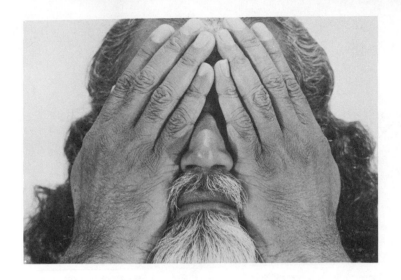

Cupping the Eyes

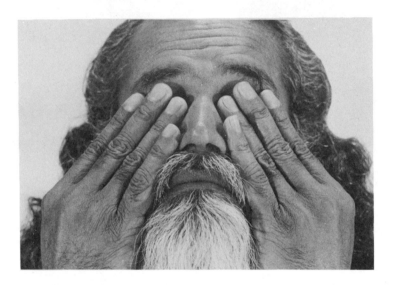

Massaging the Eyes

After completing the exercises, close the eyes. Rub the palms together rapidly until they feel quite warm. Then cup the eyes with the palms, without pressing the palms against the eyes. Feel the darkness and let your eyes absorb the warmth. When the eyes are fully relaxed, slowly bring the palms down over the cheeks until the fingertips reach the closed eyelids. Gently move the fingertips to the outer edges of the eyes, with a gentle, massaging motion, and bring the hands down.

C A U T I O N : Do not strain your eyes. Make sure that your head does not move during these exercises, just your eyes.
B E N E F I T S : All of the eye muscles are exercised. It helps to increase the circulation, tones the optic nerves, and is a general aid to the improvement of the eyesight.

II

These exercises are completely different from those given in Nethra Vyāyāmam-Section I. In Section I there is movement of the eyes, but here they remain steady, gazing at a particular point. They are being given here only because they are concerned with the eyes. However, they should be practiced at a different time and should be considered as part of the exercises mentioned in Thratakam (page 176).

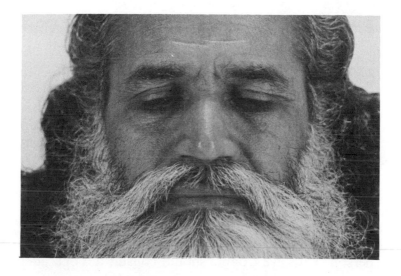

NĀSĀGRA DRISHTI—(*Ex. 1*)

EXERCISE 1: *Nāsāgra Drishti*. Gently bring the gaze toward the tip of the nose. Continue gazing as long as can be comfortably done.

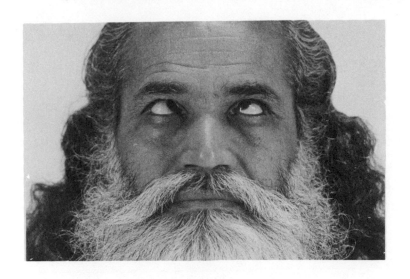

BRUMADHYA DRISHTI—(*Ex. 2*)

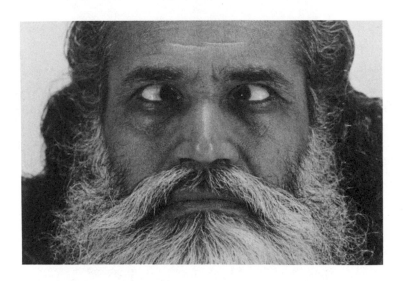

MADHYAMA DRISHTI—(*Ex. 3*)

EXERCISE 2: *Brumadhya Drishti.* Gently bring the gaze toward the space between the eyebrows. Continue gazing as long as can be comfortably done.

EXERCISE 3: *Madhyama Drishti.* Gently bring the gaze toward the root of the nose. Continue gazing as long as can be comfortably done.

CAUTION: Avoid any undue strain to the eyes. Practice these exercises slowly and cautiously. Those persons with eye trouble should consult a Yoga adept before starting this practice.

BENEFITS: These exercises help to improve the eyesight and aid in developing concentration.

PART TWO

SOORYA NAMASKĀRAM
or
SALUTATION TO THE SUN

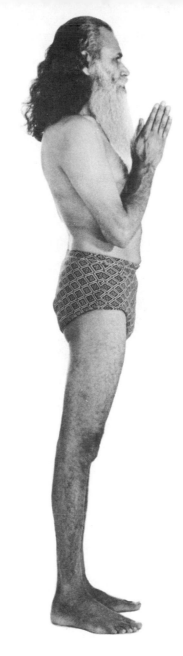

The traditional way of practicing Soorya Namaskāram is to get up early in the morning and, after the morning routine of a bowel movement and washing, to stand facing the sun, performing the poses with an attitude of worship. This doesn't mean that Soorya Namaskāram should be practiced only at this time. Any time that is good for practicing Yoga āsanas is a good time to do Soorya Namaskāram.

TECHNIQUE: There are twelve positions in each round of Soorya Namaskāram. These are as follows:

Position 1: Stand erect with the feet together. The palms should be touching each other, opposite the middle of the chest, fingers pointing upward.

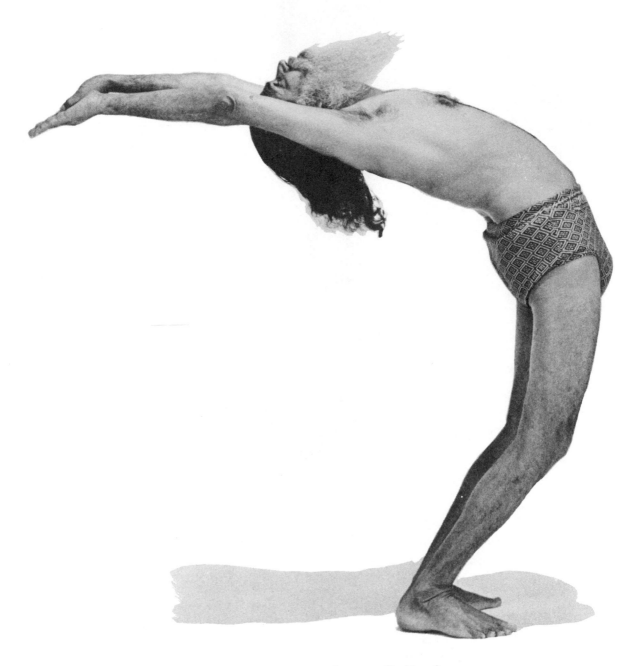

SOORYA NAMASKĀRAM—*Position 2*

Position 2: Raise the arms over the head, locking the thumbs and keeping the arms alongside the ears. Bend backward, looking up at the hands, with feet firmly planted.

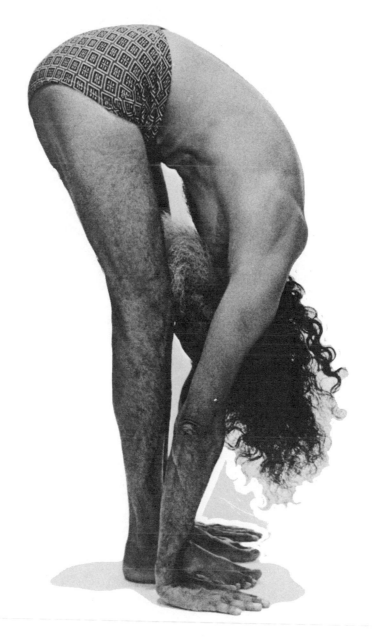

SOORYA NAMASKĀRAM—*Position 3*

Position 3: Keeping the head between the arms, bend forward, trying to place the palms flat on the floor on either side of the feet. The knees should be kept straight. Try to bring the face to the knees.

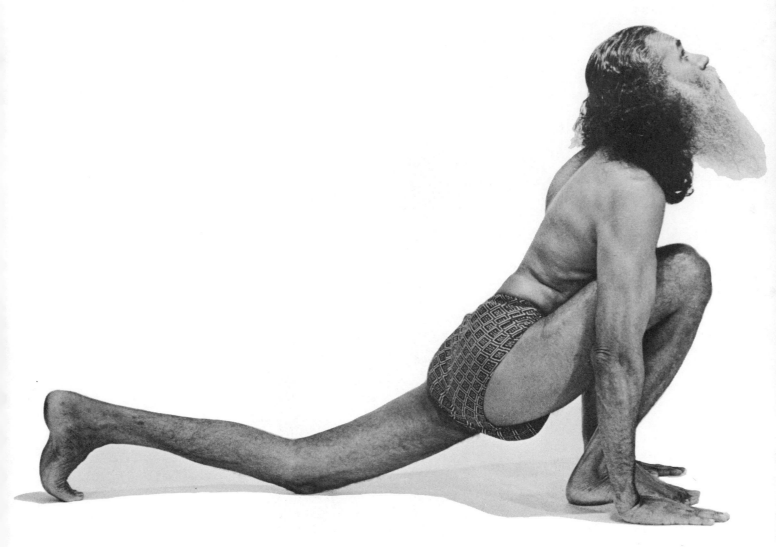

SOORYA NAMASKĀRAM—*Position 4*

Position 4: Stretch the left leg back, bringing the left knee to the floor. The right foot remains between the hands, the right knee touching the chest. Look up.

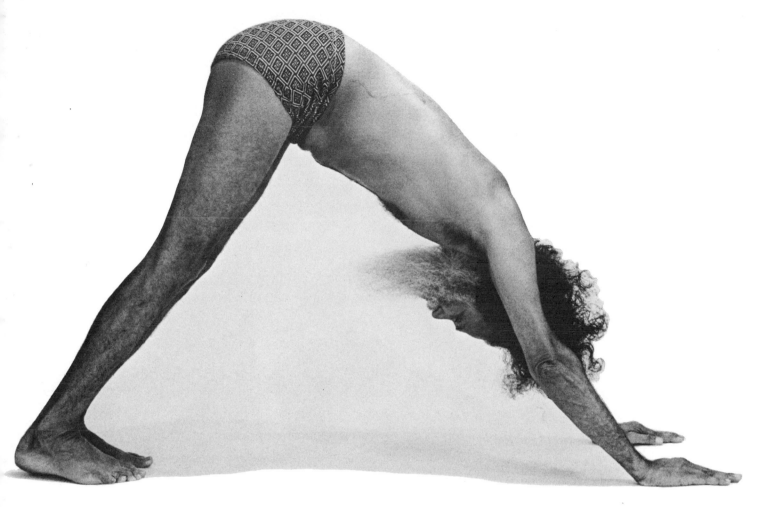

SOORYA NAMASKĀRAM—*Position 5*

Position 5: Bring the right leg back to meet the left foot. The body now forms an arch, with the head between the arms and the heels stretching toward the floor. Look at the feet.

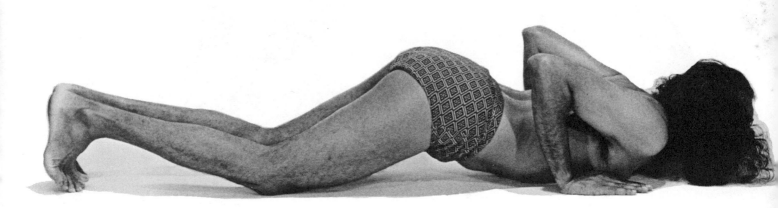

SOORYA NAMASKĀRAM—*Position 6*

Position 6:   In succession, bring the knees to the floor, the chest to the floor, the chin to the floor. The pelvis should remain slightly off the floor. The palms are now beneath the shoulders.

[16   ]

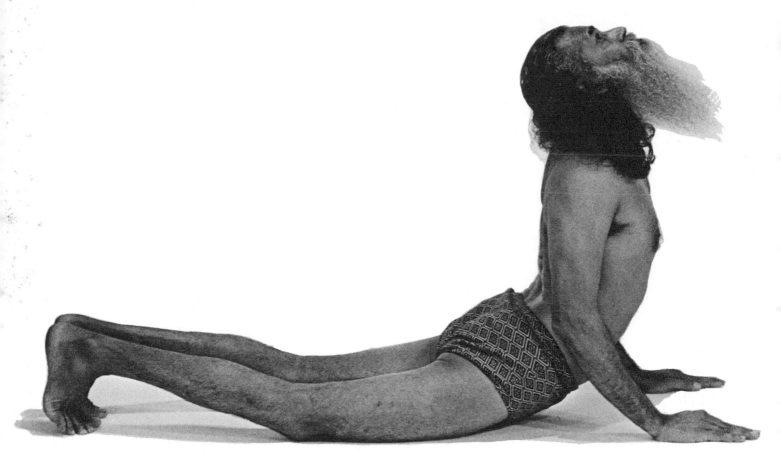

SOORYA NAMASKĀRAM—*Position 7*

Position 7: Bringing the pelvis to the floor, stretch up the head, neck, and chest, looking at the ceiling as in Bhujangāsana (cobra pose). The elbows remain alongside the body, slightly bent so that the weight rests on the back.

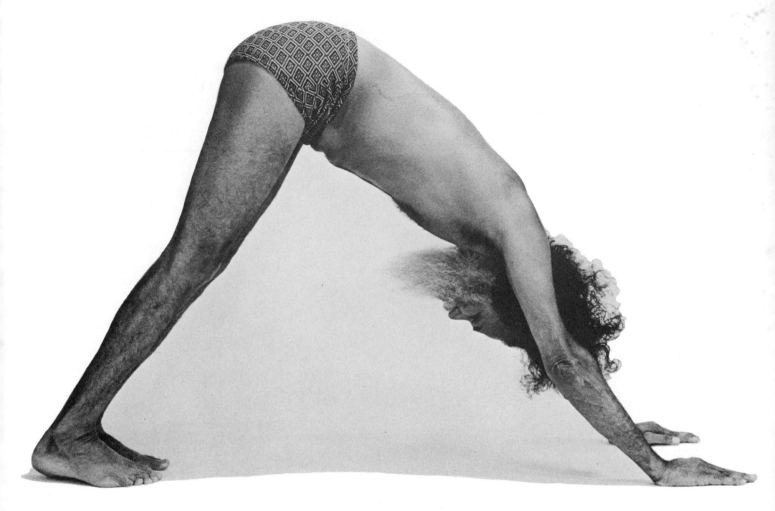

SOORYA NAMASKĀRAM—*Position 8*

Position 8: In one movement, bring the head between the arms, raising the body into an arch, as in Position 5, stretching the heels toward the floor.

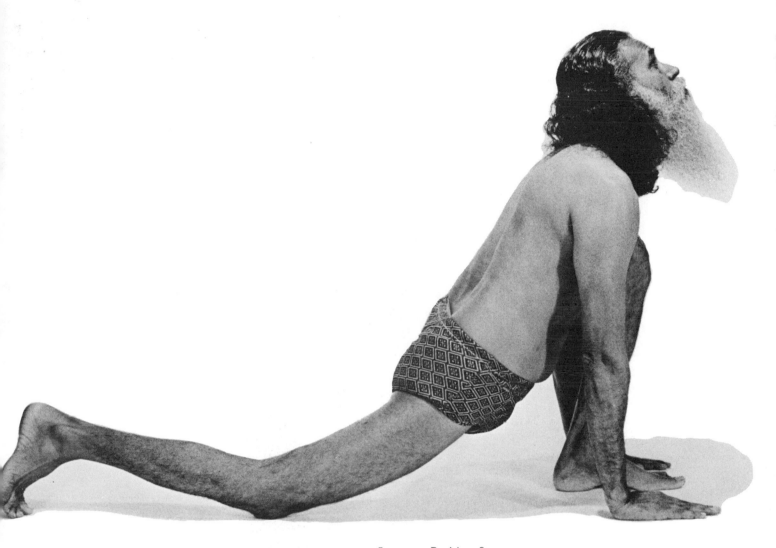

SOORYA NAMASKĀRAM—*Position 9*

Position 9:   Thrust the left leg forward between the hands, with the left knee touching the chest. The right leg is now stretched back, with the right knee touching the floor. Look up. This position is the reverse of Position 4.

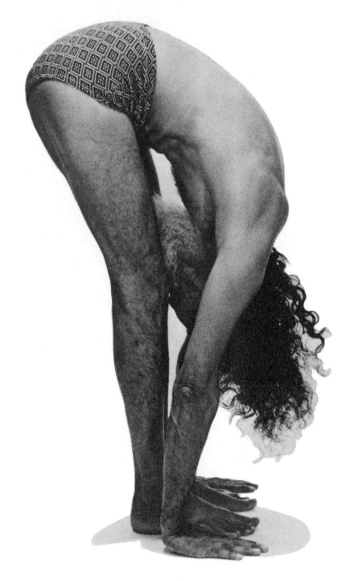

SOORYA NAMASKĀRAM—*Position 10*

Position 10: Bringing the right leg forward, straighten out the knees. Try to place the palms flat on the floor on either side of the feet. Try to bring the face to the knees, as in Position 3.

[20]

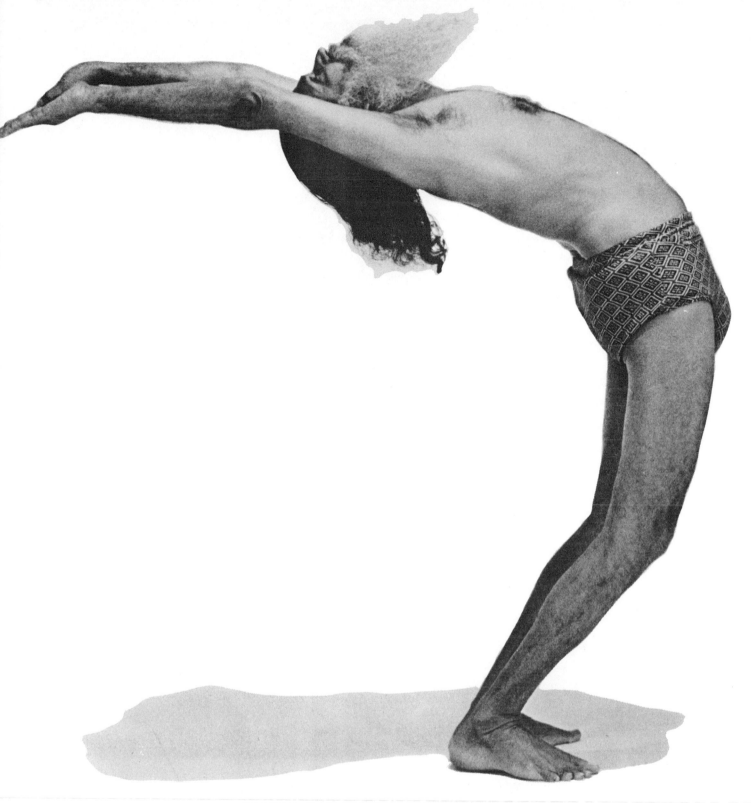

SOORYA NAMASKĀRAM—*Position 11*

Position 11: Keeping the arms alongside the ears, stretch up and back, looking at the hands, as in Position 2.

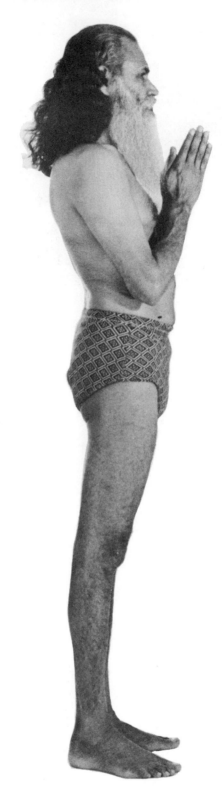

SOORYA NAMASKĀRAM—*Position 12*

Position 12:   Bring the arms down, bring the palms together, opposite the middle of the chest, stand erect, as in Position 1.

[22]

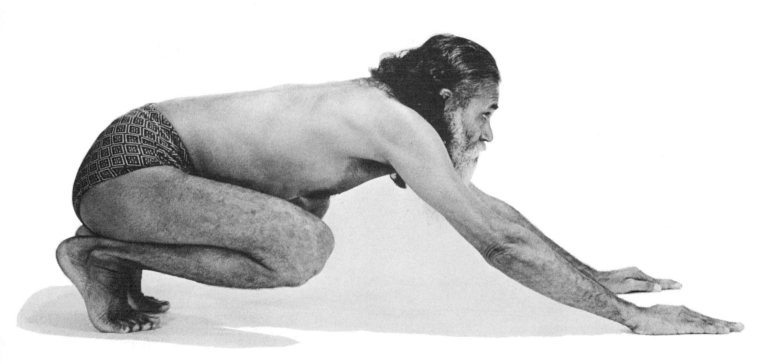

SOORYA NAMASKĀRAM—*Dip-Advanced Position 6*

VARIATION: Advanced students may use a technique known as "The Dip" in Position 6 and 7.

Advanced Position 6:   From the arch in Position 5, bring the body back in a squat position, with the buttocks touching the heels, the balance on the toes, and the knees touching the chest.

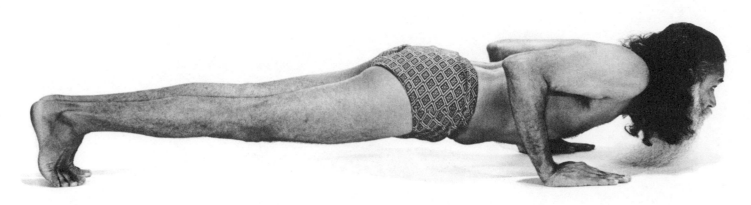

SOORYA NAMASKĀRAM—*Dip-Advanced Position 7*

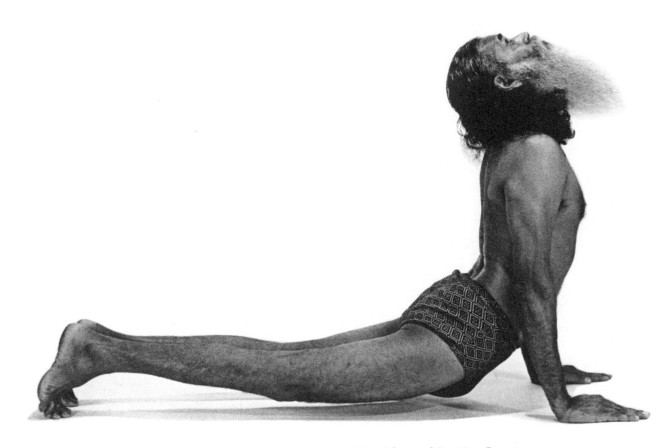

SOORYA NAMASKĀRAM—*Dip-Advanced Position 7*

Advanced Position 7: In one movement, thrust the body forward, parallel to but not touching the floor. When the shoulders come to a point above the palms, stretch the head, neck and chest up to look at the ceiling, as in Bhujangāsana (cobra pose). However, in this position, the body is not touching the floor. Then go on to the regular Position 8.

[24]

CAUTION: The position of the feet in 1, 2, and 3 will be the same in 10, 11, and 12. From Positions 4 through 9, the hands will take over that same position. You should end up in the exact position you started. *Do not overexert yourself.*

BREATHING: Exhale on Position 1, inhale on 2, exhale on 3, inhale on 4, exhale on 5, inhale on 6, hold the breath on 7, exhale on 8, inhale on 9, exhale on 10, inhale on 11, exhale on 12.

TIME: According to your own capacity, gradually increase the number of Soorya Namaskārams.

BENEFITS: Soorya Namaskāram has a beneficial influence over the entire personality, as it is a very complete combination of bodily postures and breathing, plus the prayerful attitude of the mind. To quiet the restless mind, Soorya Namaskāram can be done slowly. If, however, the mind is in a dull, lazy, or drowsy state, Soorya Namaskāram can be performed quite rapidly, almost like a physical drill. This will bring alertness to the mind. Hence, Soorya Namaskāram is a general tonic.

NOTE: The king of Oundh, India (formerly Ayodhya), after understanding the benefit of Soorya Namaskāram, taught it to his queen and together they demonstrated it throughout their state, making it a compulsory part of physical training programs in the schools. No wonder that entire state enjoyed perfect health and harmony!

"Modern life is exceedingly wearing; the noise, the excitement, the hurry, the competition, irregular hours, hard study, anxieties, worry, lack of proper food and exercise make a heavy tax on the constitution soon resulting in a breakdown of health. One can, however, be unaffected by these evils of modern civilization, if one should perform the Soorya Namaskar exercise daily and take care of the diet, and make proper use of sunshine and open air."

—THE KING OF AUNDH (India, 1940)

PART THREE

MEDITATIVE POSES

As mentioned in the Introduction, the Sage Pathanjali defines "āsana" as one that gives steadiness and comfort. Such an āsana is very necessary for deep meditation, because at that time the body should neither be a hindrance nor a burden on the mind, and should be easily forgotten.

This comfort can be attained by any one of the foregoing sitting postures. For in them, the body will find its own center of gravity, so that you can easily transcend it to dwell in the mental realm for any length of time.

Keeping the spine in a vertical position helps the nerve current to flow through the different nerve centers and awaken the psychic forces.

Therefore, select any one of the meditative poses suitable to you and learn to sit in it. Begin sitting in it for five or ten minutes and gradually increase that period. Very soon you may find that even two or three hours of sitting does not tire you, but rather you will enjoy sitting even longer. At that time you will see how much easier your meditation becomes.

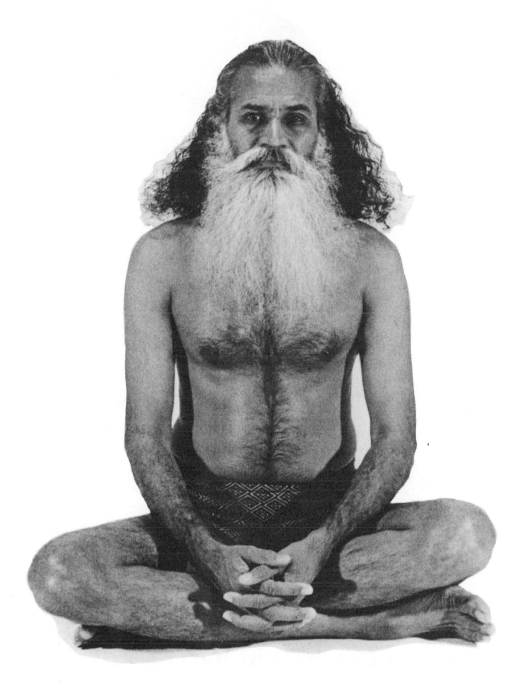

SUKHĀSANA

1 / SUKHĀSANA OR THE COMFORTABLE POSE

TECHNIQUE: Sit with the legs stretched forward. Comfortably cross the legs under the thighs. Keep the hands folded in front of the body.

BENEFITS: This pose is good for those who find it difficult to sit in other meditative poses.

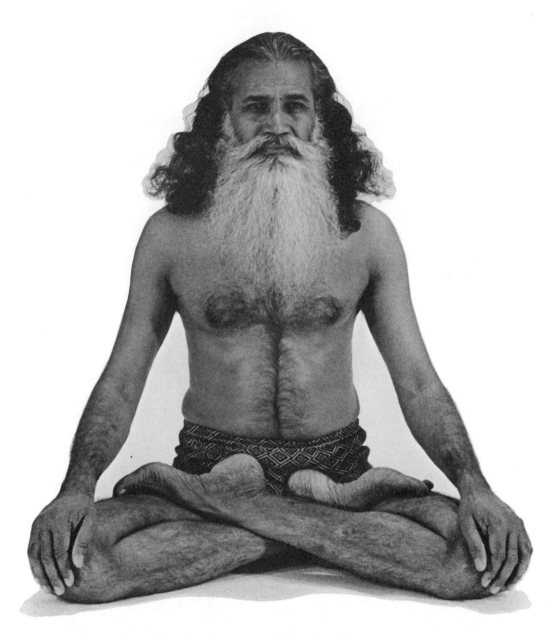

PADMĀSANA—*Palms Turned Down*

2 / PADMĀSANA OR THE LOTUS POSE

TECHNIQUE:
Stage I: The first stage of Padmāsana is Arddha Padmāsana (half lotus). Sit with the legs stretched forward. Rest the right foot on the left thigh with the sole turned up. Let the right knee touch the floor. Fold the left leg, so that the left heel rests under the right thigh. Stretch out the arms, resting the wrists against the corresponding knees, palms turned down, or turn the palms up in Chin Mudra (*see* Chin Mudra) with the index fingers touching the thumbs. Keep the head, neck, and trunk of the body in a straight line. Breathe normally.
Stage II: When you can easily do Stage I, you can begin to practice full Padmāsana. Again sit with the legs stretched forward. Rest the right foot on the left thigh with the sole turned up. Let the right knee touch the floor. Gently fold the left leg, bringing the

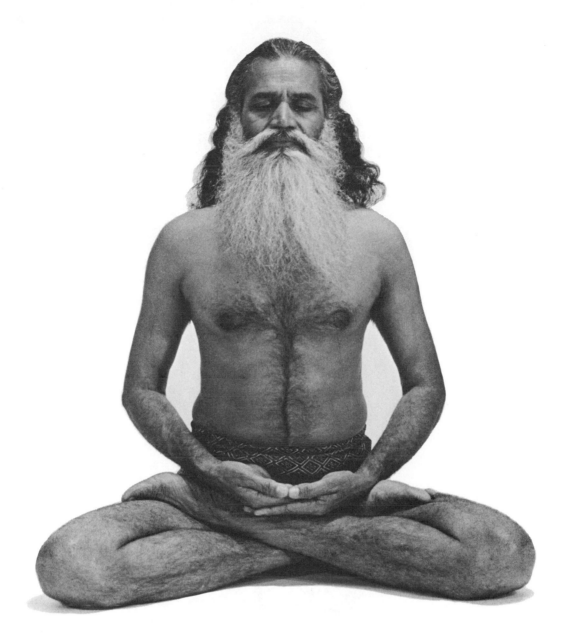

PADMĀSANA—*Palms Turned Up*

left foot to rest over the right thigh with the sole turned up. Both heels should be touching the abdomen. Place the left hand between the heels with the palm turned up. Place the right hand over the left in a similar manner or stretch out the hands as in Stage I. Keep the head, neck, and trunk in a straight line. Breathe normally.

CAUTION: The body should be relaxed and the chest well spread out. At no time should one exert or strain any part of the legs.

TIME: When Padmāsana is practiced along with other āsanas, the maximum duration should be one minute. When practiced at other times, the duration can be as long as one finds it comfortable.

BENEFITS: This pose is highly suited for meditation as well as prānāyāma. It helps increase digestion, aids good appetite, helps in removing rheumatism, and is an aid to strengthening the nerves of the legs and thighs. It helps to keep the wind, bile, and phlegm in proper proportion and is an aid in maintaining celibacy.

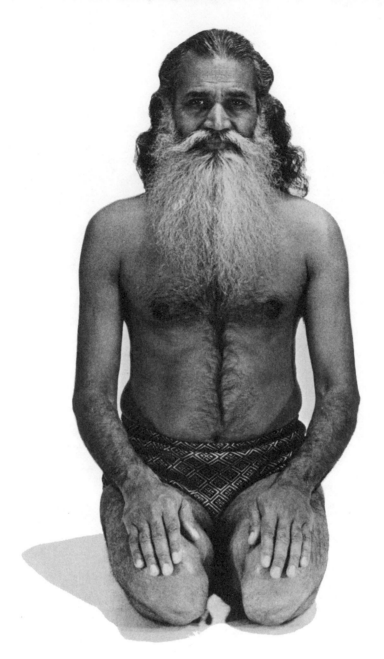

VAJRĀSANA

3 / VAJRĀSANA OR THE PELVIC POSE

TECHNIQUE: Kneel down on the floor, keeping the knees together. The entire length of the legs, from the knees to the toes, should be touching the ground. The heels should be apart, and the toes should touch. Then, slowly sit back on the legs. Keep the trunk of the body, the head, and the neck in a straight line. Place the palms over the knees. Let the major weight of the body fall on the ankles. Breathe normally.

CAUTION: The body should be relaxed and not stiff. At the beginning of practice

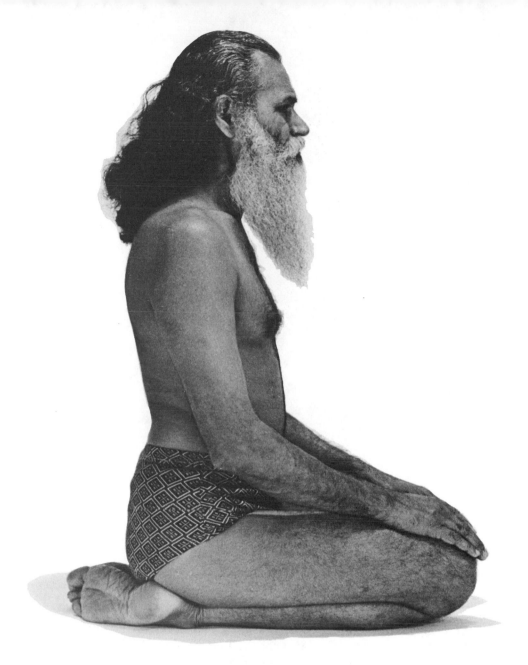

VAJRĀSANA

of Vajrāsana there may be a slight pain near the knees and ankles, but it will soon pass away.

TIME: As in Padmāsana.

BENEFITS: This pose is useful if practiced as a meditation pose. (It is used so by many.) If done immediately after eating, it aids digestion. It gives firmness and strength to the muscles of the legs and thighs. It helps relieve flatulence (gas), indigestion, sciatica, and dyspepsia. It stimulates the most vital part (konda, in the Yogic language) situated behind the navel pit, and tones up the entire nervous system. It also helps in the cure of elephantiasis.

NOTE: Placing the buttocks on the floor, between the parted heels, could make a variation in Vajrāsana.

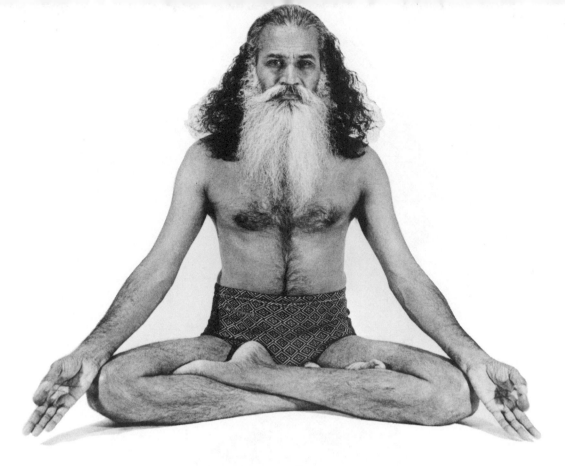

SWASTIKĀSANA

4 / SWASTIKĀSANA OR THE FAVORABLE POSE

TECHNIQUE: Sit with the legs stretched forward. Bend one leg (for convenience, the right will be used as an example) and set the heel against the left groin with the right sole touching the left thigh. Then, bend the left leg and bring the left heel close to the right groin, after crossing over the right ankle and bringing the left sole to touch the right thigh. Gently insert the left toes between the right thigh and calf, with only the big toe visible. From below, insert the right toes between the left thigh and calf, pulling the big toe up and out so that it looks the same as the big toe of the left foot. Keep the trunk of the body, the head, and the neck in a straight line. The arms may rest with the wrists against the knees and palms, or in Chin Mudra form.

CAUTION: Adjust the crossing position of the ankles conveniently so that there is no undue pressure on the bones.

TIME: As in Padmāsana.

BENEFITS: This pose is good for longer meditations, particularly for those who do not find Padmāsana or Siddhāsana easy.

NOTE: The crossing of two lines at right angles to each other, according to the beliefs of both East and West, represents auspiciousness or favorable conditions. As the legs cross each other at the ankles in this pose, it is known as Swastika (favorable) āsana.

[34]

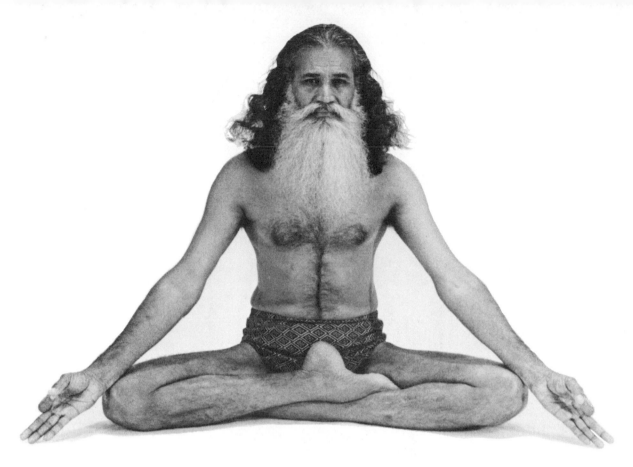

SIDDHĀSANA

5 / SIDDHĀSANA OR THE ACCOMPLISHED POSE

TECHNIQUE: Sit with the legs stretched forward. Bend the left leg and place the heel against the perineum—just below the genitals. The left sole should touch the right thigh closely. Avoid sitting on the heel. Then, bend the right leg also, placing the right heel against the pubic bone, a little above the genitals. The right sole should closely touch the left thigh, with the toes tucked in between the left thigh and calf. Keep the trunk of the body, the neck, and the head in a straight line. The arms may be stretched out, with the wrists against the corresponding knees and the palms turned down. This pose may be practiced in combination with Chin Mudra, Jālandhra Bandha and Moola Bandha (see Parts Six and Seven). Breathe normally throughout this pose.

CAUTION: Good care must be taken to prevent hurting the genitals while placing the heels in position. The body should be relaxed. Only men should practice Siddhāsana. Women interested in this pose should seek the advice of a Yoga adept.

TIME: When Siddhāsana is practiced along with other āsanas, the maximum duration should be one minute. When practiced at other times, the duration can be as long as one finds it comfortable.

BENEFITS: This pose is very helpful for meditation. Those who find Padmāsana difficult will find Siddhāsana more convenient to practice. It tones the entire abdominal viscera and sexual glands. It helps in sexual control as well.

NOTE: Some claim that Siddhāsana adversely affects the sexual powers, but there is no evidence to prove this.

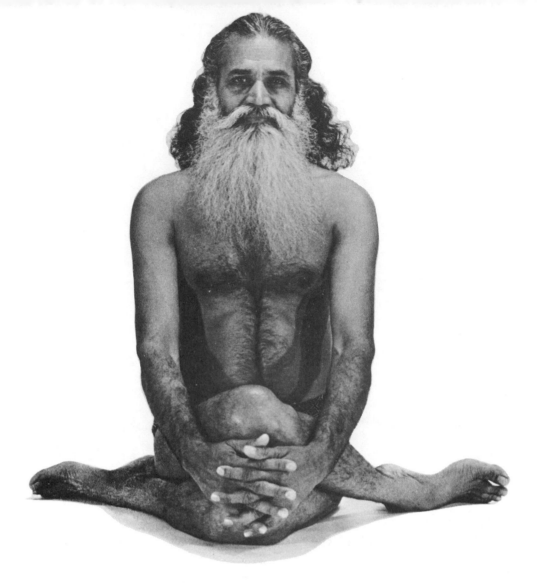

VEERĀSANA

6 / VEERĀSANA OR THE HEROIC POSE

TECHNIQUE: Sit on the floor and fold back the left leg so that it lies outside the right buttock, with the left heel pressing close against the right thigh. Then, cross the right leg over the left and take the right heel back so that it lies outside the left thigh. If the right heel cannot touch the left thigh, it does not matter. The right knee will be raised somewhat. Interlock the hands and place them, palms facing inward, between the knees. The left knee, the interlocked fingers, and the right knee should all be in one straight line, one above the other. Sit straight, keeping the trunk of the body, the head, and the neck in a straight line.

CAUTION: In this āsana, avoid hurting the genitals and testes as the thighs are brought close together.

TIME: As in Padmāsana.

BENEFITS: The noteworthy effects of this pose are on the gonads, or sex glands. It helps to maintain good control over the sex impulse and will give great benefit to the sexually weak or those who are interested in strict celibacy.

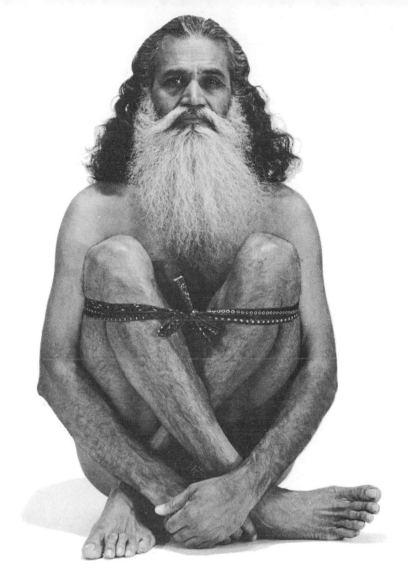

YOGA BATTĀSANA

7 / YOGA BATTĀSANA OR THE YOGIC BELT POSE

TECHNIQUE: Sit with the legs stretched forward. Cross the legs and bring the knees up against the chest. Sit straight. Tie the trunk and legs together with a soft belt or sash.

BENEFITS: Tying the belt around the trunk and legs will help you to keep the spine erect. Those who find it difficult to bring the knees down in a cross-legged position will find this pose useful.

NOTE: Once you have made the knot on the belt, and have found it suitable, retain the loop in that position for future use.

PART FOUR

CULTURAL POSES

I

These poses are practiced mainly as an aid to gaining perfect health. The poses given in this section are for those people interested in practicing a minimum number of poses to gain the maximum amount of benefit.

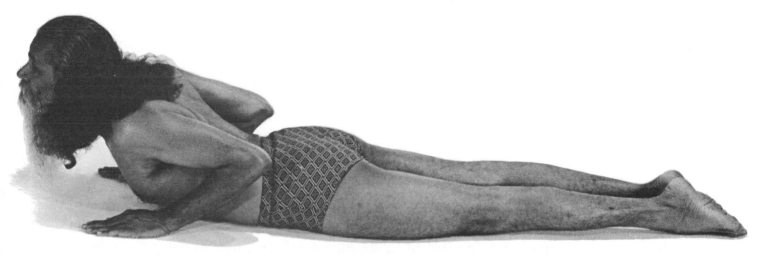

BHUJANGĀSANA—*Figure 1*

1 / BHUJANGĀSANA OR THE COBRA POSE

TECHNIQUE: Lie face downward with the forehead touching the floor. Relax all the muscles completely. Place the palms on the floor, below the corresponding shoulders, with the elbows raised and close to the trunk of the body. Keep the legs close together on the floor, with the toes pointed. Now slowly raise the head and bend the neck as far backward as possible. Only after this has been done do you slowly raise the chest

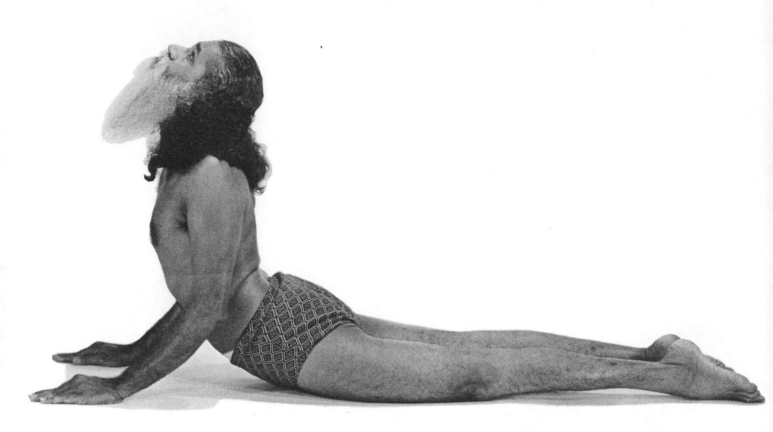

BHUJANGĀSANA—*Figure 2*

also, bending the vertebrae backward one by one. The lower part of the body, from navel to toes, should be touching the floor. Look up and behind you as far as possible. Stay this way awhile and then come down, lowering the trunk first, then the head—very slowly—to the ground. Inhale while rising, breathe normally while retaining the pose, and exhale while coming down.

CAUTION: Do not raise the body suddenly, with a jerk. Try to pull the chest up with the help of the back muscles, rather than allowing the weight to fall on the hands. Avoid the tendency to breathe through the mouth.

TIME: Repeat three to six times, retaining the pose for ten seconds at a time. Gradually reduce this repetition and try to retain the pose just once for a maximum duration of one minute.

BENEFITS: In this pose, the back muscles are exercised and gain in health. The spine becomes elastic and the chest expands. The cranial nerves are exercised to maintain their activity and tone for a long time. Any slight displacement of the spinal column gets adjusted. Backache caused by overwork, constipation, and flatulence (gas) is relieved. In women, the ovaries and uterus are toned up; various utero-ovarial complaints are relieved.

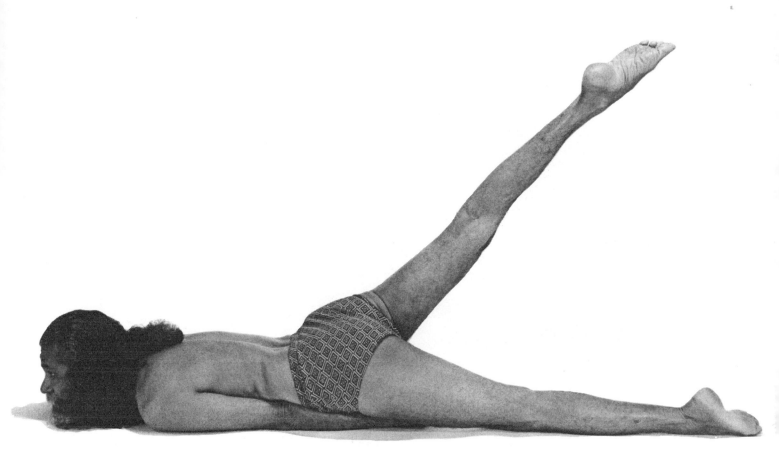

ARDDHA SALABĀSANA

2 / ARDDHA SALABĀSANA OR THE HALF LOCUST POSE

TECHNIQUE: Lie face downward with the chin against the floor. Tuck the arms underneath the body, with the palms upward, underneath the thighs. Try to make the elbows touch. Keep the toes pointed. Inhale, retaining the breath, stiffen the body, and raise the right leg, without bending the knee. Allow the entire weight to rest on the chest and arms. Slowly lower the leg and exhale slowly. Relax. Then do the same with the left leg.

When you are well used to this pose, do the full pose, or Salabāsana (please see next pose).

TIME: Repeat each leg, alternating, twice.

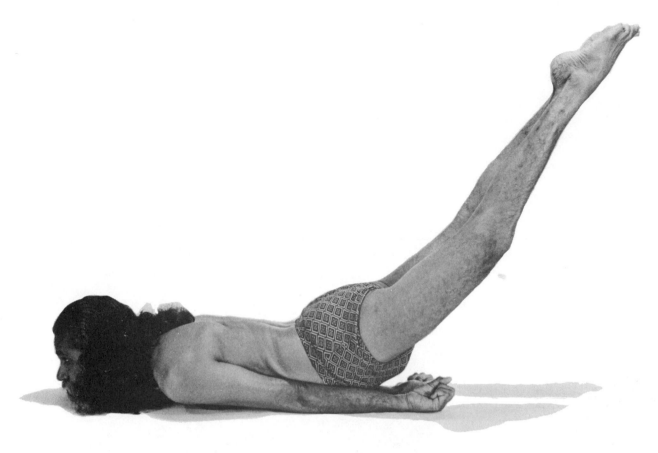

SALABĀSANA

3 / SALABĀSANA OR THE LOCUST POSE

TECHNIQUE: Lie face downward with the chin against the floor. Tuck the arms underneath the body, with the palms upward, underneath the thighs. Try to make the elbows touch. Keep the toes pointed. Inhale, retaining the breath, stiffen the body, and raise both legs, without bending the knees. Allow the entire weight to rest on the chest and arms. Maintain the pose for as long as you can comfortably retain the breath. Slowly lower the legs, exhale slowly, and relax.

CAUTION: After a certain amount of practice, this pose may be retained while breathing normally. Before repeating the pose, pause sufficiently to bring the breathing back to normal.

NOTE: Intermediate and advanced students of āsanas may begin this pose by lying face downward, chin against the floor, with the arms alongside the body, palms facing upward and fists clenched.

TIME: Repeat three to six times, retaining the pose for ten seconds at a time. Gradually reduce this repetition and try to retain the pose just once for a maximum duration of one minute.

BENEFITS: In this pose the back, pelvis, and abdomen are exercised. The sympathetic nervous system is toned up. It helps to relieve sluggishness of the liver and the pains of lumbago.

[44]

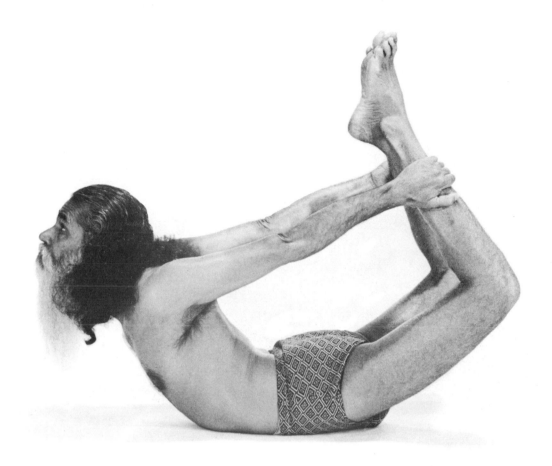

DHANURĀSANA

4 / DHANURĀSANA OR THE BOW POSE

TECHNIQUE: Lie face downward, with the forehead against the floor. Gently fold the legs back and hold the ankles with the corresponding hands. Raise the head, chest, and thighs, arching the back and allowing the entire weight of the body to fall on the abdomen. Inhale while rising, breathe normally while retaining pose, and exhale while coming down.

CAUTION: Do not pull the legs up by bending the elbows. Let the arms be straight. Pull the legs up only enough to raise the thighs off the floor. Persons suffering from high blood pressure, hernia, or an ulcer either in the stomach or intestines should avoid this pose.

TIME: Repeat three to six times, retaining the pose for ten seconds at a time. Gradually reduce this repetition and try to retain the pose just once for a maximum duration of one minute.

BENEFITS: This pose gives all the benefits gained by practicing Bhujangāsana (cobra pose) and Salabāsana (locust pose). In addition, it reduces abdominal fat, increases the peristaltic movement of the bowels, and tones up the pancreas, thus helping to cure diabetes. This āsana is of special benefit to women.

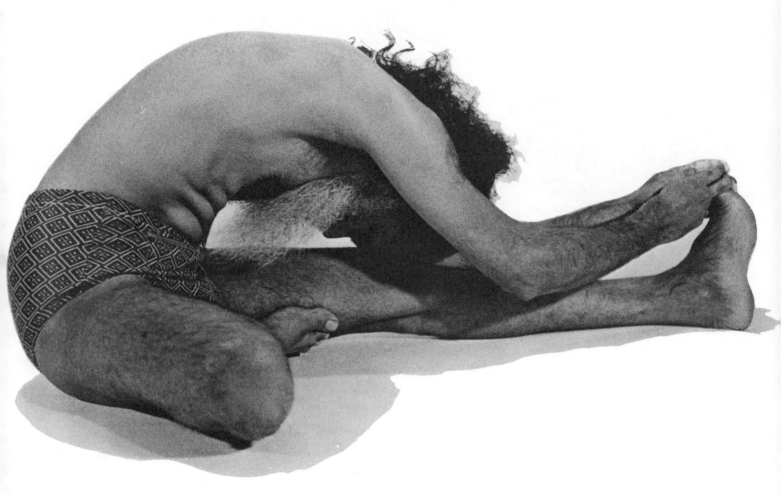

JĀNUSIRSHĀSANA

5 / JĀNUSIRSHĀSANA OR THE HEAD-TO-KNEE POSE

TECHNIQUE: Sit on the floor with both legs stretched forward. Bend the left leg, bringing the heel against the body. Feel the pressure on the anus. Bend forward as much as possible, grasping the right toe with both hands. Retain the pose as long as you can comfortably do so. Repeat the pose, bending the right leg.

Variation: Placing the heel over the opposite thigh, rather than against the body, is another variation of Jānusirshāsana.

TIME: Repeat two to three times on each leg, retaining the pose for ten seconds at a time. Gradually reduce this and try to retain the pose just once on each leg for a maximum duration of one minute.

BENEFITS: This pose helps to control the sexual energy and to maintain celibacy for those interested. It also helps in evacuating the bowels.

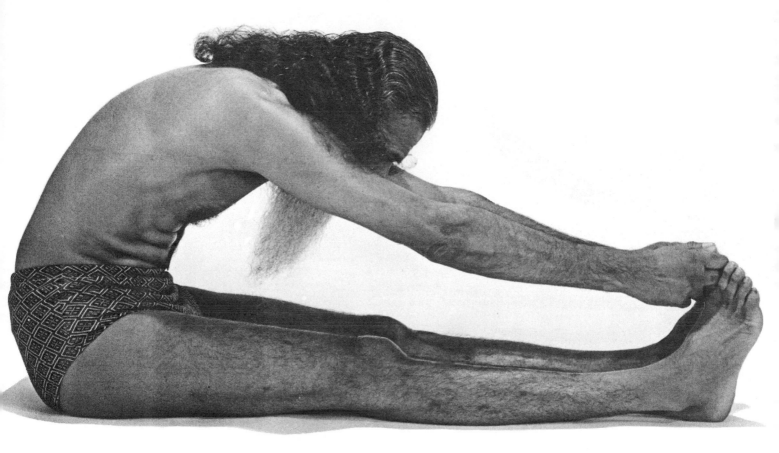

PASCHIMOTHĀNĀSANA—*Figure 1*

6 / PASCHIMOTHĀNĀSANA, THE POSTERIOR-STRETCHING POSE OR THE FORWARD-BENDING POSE

TECHNIQUE:

Stage I: Lie flat on the back. Stretch the arms over the head and alongside the floor, locking the thumbs. The upper arms should almost touch the ears. Stiffen the entire body, holding the breath, and slowly raise the arms, head, and chest simultaneously, assuming a sitting position, with the arms stretched over the head. See that the arms do not descend and that the legs do not jerk upward as you rise. After this, slowly bend forward, exhaling, and hold on to the big toes with the index fingers and thumbs of the corresponding hands. Retain the pose while breathing normally.

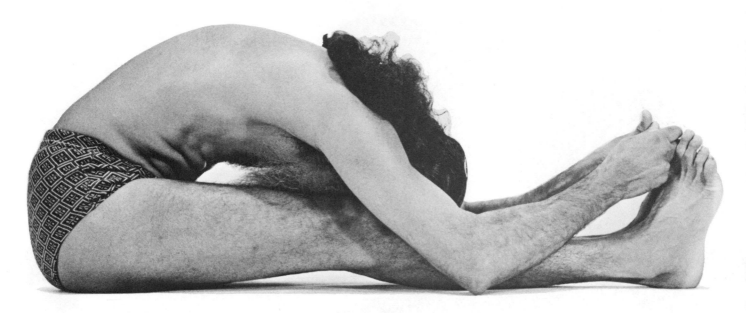

PASCHIMOTHĀNĀSANA—*Figure 2*

Stage II: Little by little, try to bring the face toward the knees, to eventually bury the face between them. The elbows should be bent, touching the floor on the outside of either leg. After a while, slowly rise and come back to the lying position on the floor. While coming back to the floor, try to keep the legs on the floor and the arms in the overhead position.

CAUTION: Do not allow the knees to bend. There should be no strain throughout the pose. If you find it difficult to sit up from a lying position, the pose may be done from a sitting position. If the toes cannot be reached at first, the legs may be held at any easily reachable place—the calves or ankles. Persons suffering from any disease of the abdominal viscera, enlargement of liver or spleen, should avoid this pose. Do not practice this pose for long if you are constipated, as it may increase this condition rather than cure it. Paschimothānāsana done for a short period will cure constipation.

TIME: Repeat three to six times, retaining the pose for ten seconds at a time. Gradually reduce this repetition and try to retain the pose just once for a maximum duration of one minute.

BENEFITS: This is an excellent stretching pose. It exercises nearly all posterior muscles and tones up the abdominal viscera. It helps in curing piles, constipation, and diabetes. It reduces potbelly and nocturnal emissions and prevents menstrual disorders.

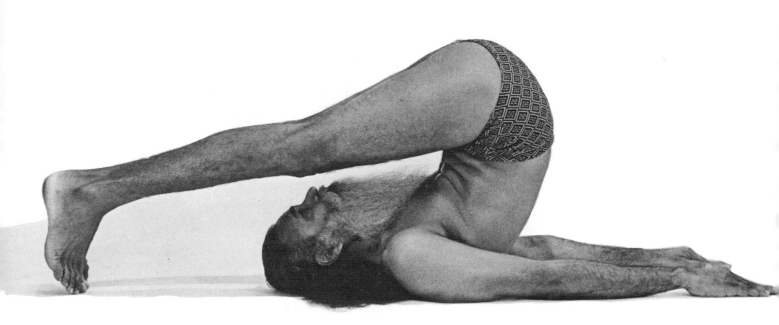

HALĀSANA

7 / HALĀSANA OR THE PLOW POSE

TECHNIQUE: Lie flat on the back, keeping the hands alongside the body. Holding the breath, slowly raise the legs—without bending the knees—pressing the palms firmly against the floor. When the legs are raised to approximately a 90-degree angle, raise the hips and the lower part of the back, bringing the legs to a vertical position. Then, exhaling, slowly lower the legs over the head and touch the floor with the toes.

As variations, the toes may be kept in any of the four positions, ranging from very close to the head to very far from the head.

CAUTION: While lowering the legs over the head, special care must be taken not to shake the body too much and lose control over the legs. Never strain in bringing the toes toward the floor. If there is strain, the shoulder and neck muscles could get sprained.

Beginners need not try this pose for some time, at least until they get fully acquainted with the other preliminary postures. (Please see appendix.)

TIME: Repeat three times, retaining the pose for twenty seconds at a time, five seconds at each of the four leg variations. Gradually reduce this repetition and try to retain this pose just once for a maximum duration of 80 seconds, 20 seconds at each variation.

BENEFITS: This is one of the finest poses to gain an elastic spine and healthy nerves, the main prerequisites for keeping young. The spinal cord is toned, and Halāsana is second only to Sarvāngāsana (shoulder stand) in toning up the thyroid gland. It is beneficial in curing enlargement of the liver and spleen, as well as certain types of diabetes, neuralgia, muscular rheumatism, indigestion, constipation, and obesity.

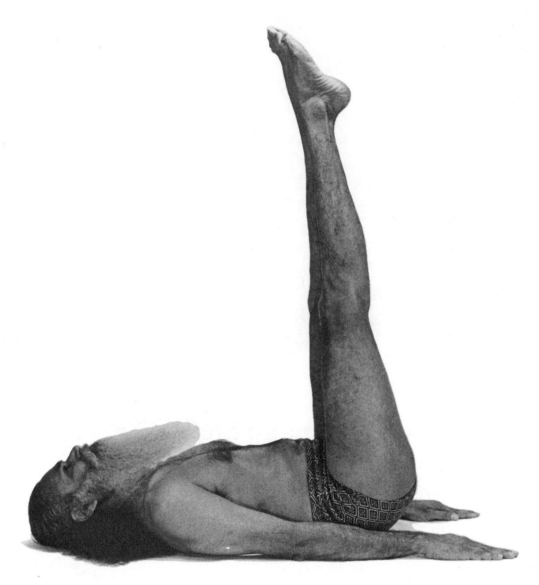

SARVĀNGĀSANA—*Figure 1*

8 / SARVĀNGĀSANA, THE ALL MEMBERS POSE OR THE SHOULDER STAND

TECHNIQUE: Lie flat on the back, placing hands alongside the body. Raise the legs up to 90 degrees. Then, raise the trunk of the body to a vertical position also, until the chin presses against the chest. As you raise the trunk, simultaneously raise the forearms (without widening or shifting the elbows) to support the back. The entire body, from neck to toes, should be as straight as possible. The back of the neck should lie flat against the floor. To come down from the pose, gently lower the legs slightly over the

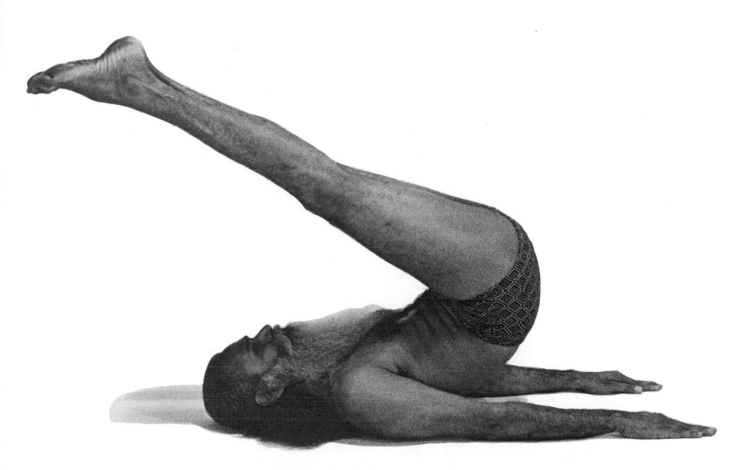

SARVĀNGĀSANA—*Figure 2*

head, thereby shifting the weight from the elbows. Replace the forearms on the floor behind the body. Bring the trunk slowly down and then the legs, not raising the head until the legs reach the floor. Breathe normally while retaining the pose. There will be a brief retention of breath while lifting the legs up and bringing them down.

CAUTION: Keep the mouth closed. If saliva collects, do not swallow it, but dispose of it after the pose is finished. If you feel like sneezing, coughing, or yawning while in the position, come down immediately, before doing so. Do not practice this pose if there is disturbance in the organs of the head or if headache or fever is present.

TIME: Repeat three times, retaining the pose for one minute to begin with. Each week add one minute to each retention, until a total period of nine minutes is reached

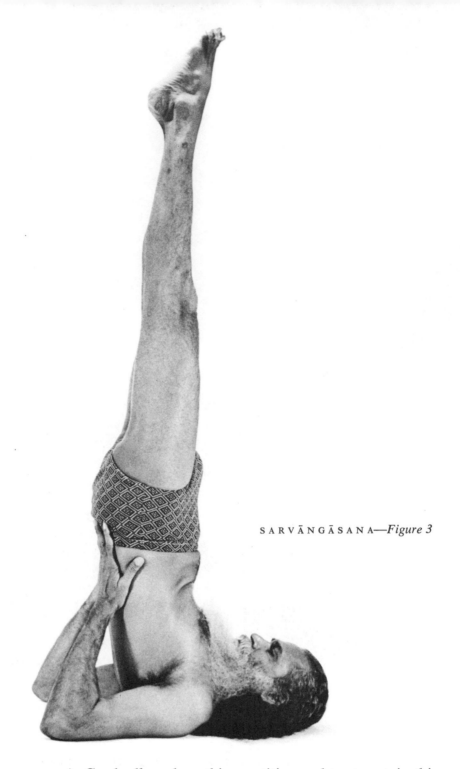

SARVĀNGĀSANA—*Figure 3*

(three minutes per pose). Gradually reduce this repetition and try to retain this pose just once for a maximum duration of ten minutes.

BENEFITS: This is an excellent pose for regulation of the sex glands, poor blood circulation, seminal weakness, and feminine disorders. It helps in curing asthma, disorders of the liver and intestines, dyspepsia, constipation, hernia, diabetes, heart troubles, urinary disorders, piles, varicose veins, and other disorders. It helps in reducing abdominal fat, and it helps in the cure of leprosy.

The name "Sarvā-Anga-Āsana" means "a beneficial pose for the whole body." This is done by toning up the most important gland—the thyroid.

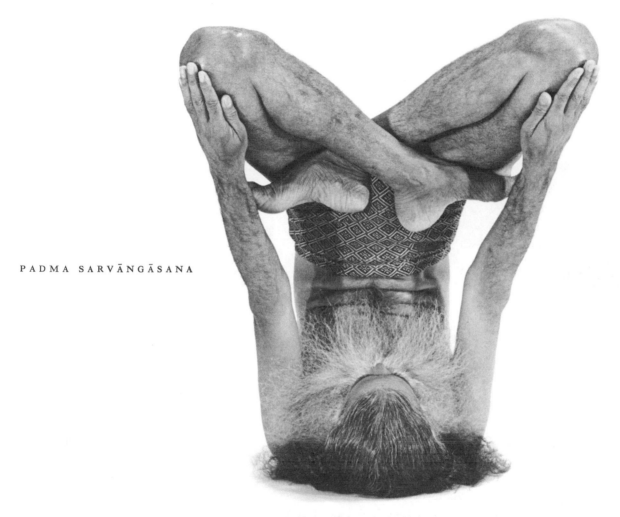

PADMA SARVĀNGĀSANA

9 / PADMA SARVĀNGĀSANA OR THE LOTUS SHOULDER STAND

TECHNIQUE: Assume Sarvāngāsana (shoulder stand). Supporting the back well, slowly fold the legs into Padmāsana (lotus pose). Maintain the pose as long as you comfortably can.

BENEFITS: This pose gives you both the benefits of Sarvāngāsana as well as those of Padmāsana.

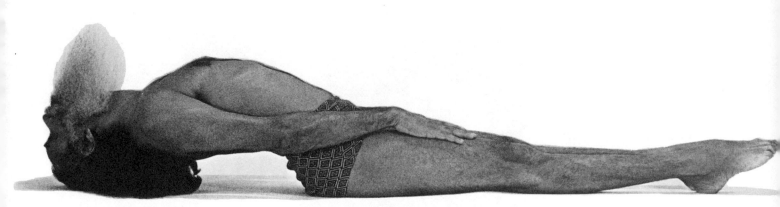

10 / MATSYĀSANA OR THE FISH POSE

TECHNIQUE: Lie flat on the floor with the palms of the hands holding the sides of the thighs. Resting the weight on the elbows, raise the head and trunk of the body. Bend the head backward, arching the spine, and place the crown of the head on the floor, creating a nice bridge between the seat and the head. Spread out the chest as much as possible and have a slight smile on the face to break up tension in the jaw. Those who have done this posture for a while can bring the palms to the tops of the thighs. While coming down, palms should again be holding the sides of the thighs. Throw the weight onto the elbows once more, lift the head off the floor, straighten the spine, and slowly come down. Deep breathing increases the benefits of the āsana, but retention of the breath is not advisable.
CAUTION: Keep the mouth closed. If saliva collects, do not swallow, but dispose of it after the pose is finished. If you feel like sneezing, coughing, or yawning, come down immediately before doing so. Do not practice this if there is disturbance in the organs of the head or if headache or fever is present.

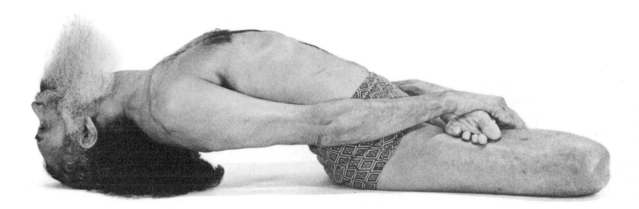

MATSYĀSANA—*Intermediate*

Do not rub the head along the floor while setting the crown on the floor or when lifting it from the floor.

TIME: Repeat two to three times, retaining this pose for fifteen seconds at a time. Gradually try to retain the pose just once for a maximum duration of two minutes.

BENEFITS: This is a complementary pose to Sarvāngāsana (shoulder stand) and relieves any cramp or stiffness in the neck caused by Sarvāngāsana. The chest cavity expands to its maximum capacity, and the apex of the lungs receives plenty of air to breathe. It helps in the prevention of asthmatic conditions, gives a natural massage to the neck and shoulders, and strengthens the waist, spine, and back muscles. It also aids in the cure of hunchback and pigeon chest.

NOTE: Intermediate and advanced students of āsanas may begin this pose by sitting in Padmāsana (lotus pose). Slowly lean backward, first on one elbow and then on the other, and lie still. Then, raise the forearms, and hold on to the toes.

Matsyāsana always follows Sarvāngāsana as a counterpose.

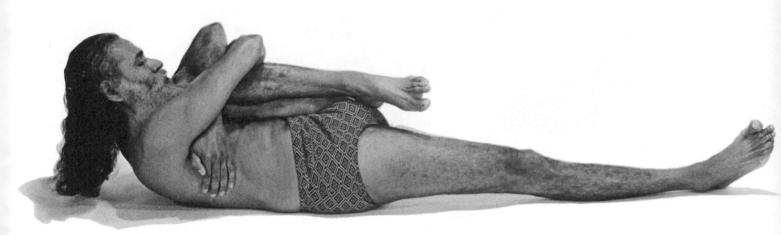

ARDDHA PAVANAMUKTĀSANA—(*Half*)

11 / PAVANAMUKTĀSANA, THE GAS-RELIEVING POSE OR THE WIND-ELIMINATING POSE

TECHNIQUE: Lie flat on the back. Raise the right leg and bend the knee, while drawing in a deep breath through the nose. Hold the breath and tightly press the knee

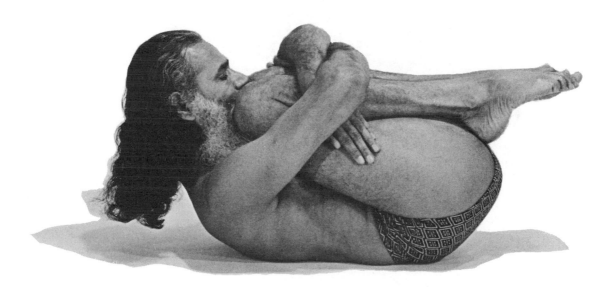

PAVANAMUKTĀSANA

against the abdomen with both hands. Raise the head and try to kiss the knee. This is Arddha (half) Pavanamuktāsana. Retain this pose as long as you can comfortably retain the breath, and then exhale slowly, coming back to the lying-down position. Repeat, using the left leg; and, finally, repeat, raising both legs in full Pavanamuktāsana.

TIME: Each stage can be repeated from three to seven times.

BENEFITS: This is an excellent pose for relieving gas in the stomach. It is an aid in toning up the abdominal viscera.

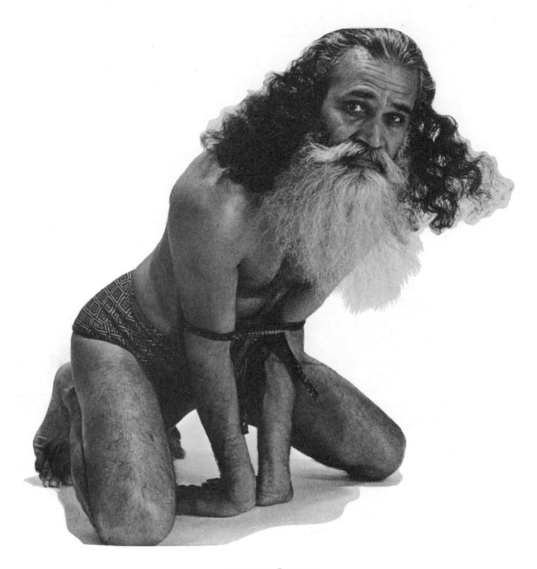

MAYURĀSANA

12 / MAYURĀSANA OR THE PEACOCK POSE

TECHNIQUE:

Stage I with Belt: Place the forearms together from the wrists to the elbows and tie with a belt. Kneel down, placing the palms together on the floor, with the fingers pointing toward the knees. There should be a forearm's length between the fingers and knees. Slowly bend the body forward, bending the arms first. The head should rest on the floor. In this position, the chest will be supported by the upper arms, and the stomach against the joined elbows. Stretch the legs, with the toes resting on the floor. Raise the head.

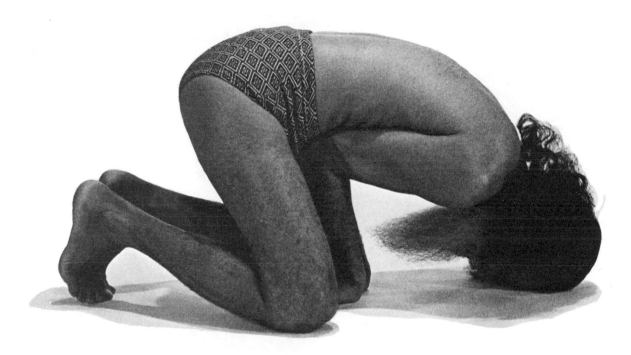

MAYURĀSANA

Stiffen the entire body like a bar resting on a fulcrum. Practice this first stage until you can do it easily, without any strain. When you can maintain this position for fifty seconds at a stretch, proceed to Stage II.

Stage II with Belt: Gently move the entire body forward with the help of the toes, thereby shifting the entire weight of the body toward the head. When the upper and lower halves of the body are in balance, the toes will automatically rise off the floor. In getting out of the posture, first place the toes on the floor and then the knees, before resuming the normal position.

Stages I and II without Belt: When your forearms are used to this pose and are well strengthened, do the pose without the aid of the belt.

C A U T I O N :   Do not jump or jerk in order to raise the legs. Avoid dashing the nose

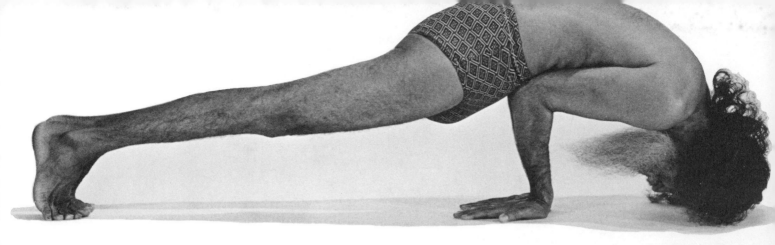

MAYURĀSANA—*Without Belt*

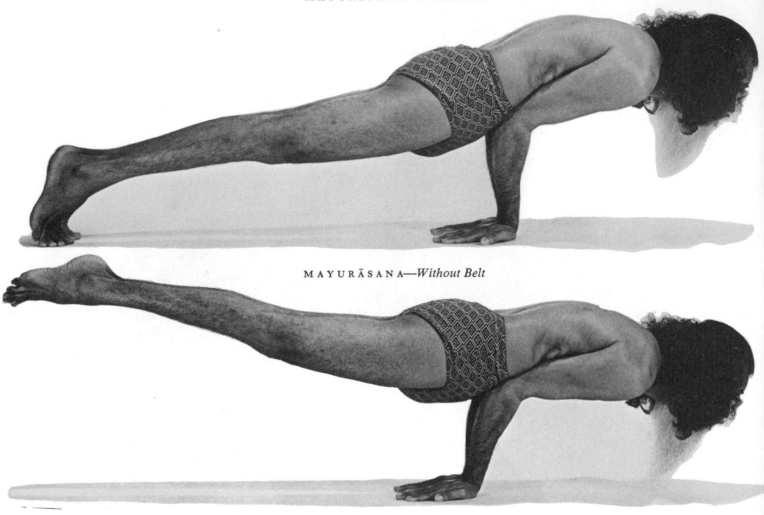

MAYURĀSANA—*Without Belt*

MAYURĀSANA—*Without Belt*

on the floor by forceful lunging or jerking. For safety's sake, place a cushion or pillow in front of the face. The wrists are greatly pressured at the beginning of this practice.

TIME: Beginners can maintain this pose from five to thirty seconds. Intermediates and advanced students can maintain it from one to two minutes.

BENEFITS: This pose braces the entire body in no time. The abdominal viscera is excellently toned up, and the pose is more or less a tonic for general health.

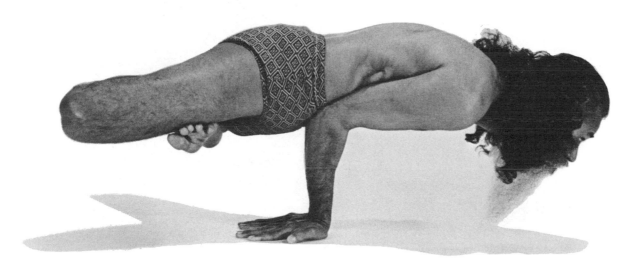

PADMA MAYURĀSANA

13 / PADMA MAYURĀSANA OR THE LOTUS PEACOCK POSE

TECHNIQUE: Assume Mayurāsana (peacock pose), and, in the final stage, when the whole body is balanced on the conjoined arms in one straight line, fold the forelegs slowly and lock them in Padmāsana (lotus pose).

CAUTION: Take care not to lose your balance while forming the lock.

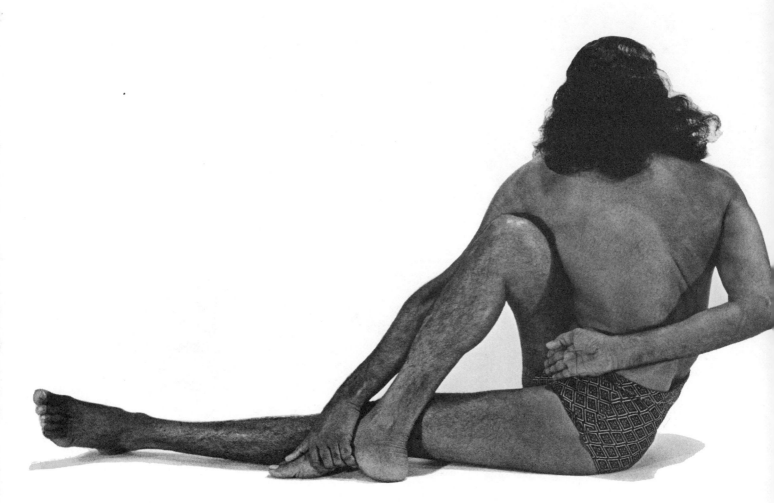

ARDDHA MATSYENDRĀSANA—*Beginners*

14 / ARDDHA MATSYENDRĀSANA OR THE HALF SPINAL TWIST

TECHNIQUE: Sit with the knees raised and the soles of the feet touching the floor about 1½ feet in front of the buttocks. Place the left leg flat on the floor. Lift the right foot and place it outside the left thigh, with the sole resting fully on the floor. The right knee should be close to the chest. Gently twist the trunk so that the left arm passes beyond the right knee and presses against it. Stretch the left arm fully to hold the left knee. Then, swing the right arm behind, twisting it clockwise around the trunk, and try to catch hold of the left thigh, in order to have the twist at the cervical vertebrae as well. Turn the head to the extreme right. Slowly come out of the pose by turning the head to the front first, then the arms and trunk, and, finally, uncrossing the legs. Bring the knees

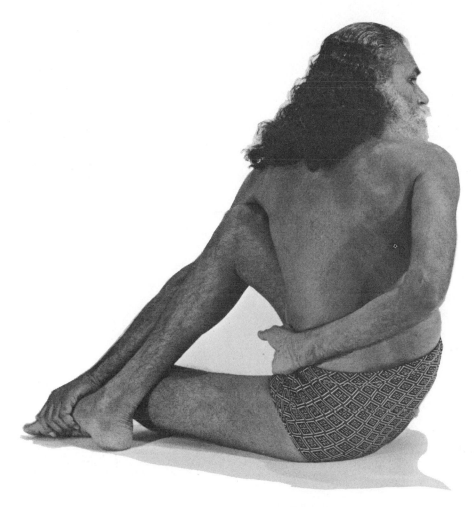

ARDDHA MATSYENDRĀSANA—*Back View*

to the raised position and then reverse the pose, using the left arm and leg. Breathe normally throughout the pose.

After a while the beginner can go on to Arddha Matsyendrāsana with the leg folded, rather than straight out in front. This is done by setting the left leg on the floor with the sole against the right thigh next to the anus. Do not rest the right buttock on the sole or allow the heel to pass outside the right thigh. After stretching the left arm fully to hold the left knee, try to stretch farther so that the left arm holds the right foot, which rests beyond the left thigh.

Variation: The right foot, which is beyond the left thigh, is taken far back and held by the right hand at the ankle. The left hand will then be holding the outside of the left knee.

CAUTION: As this pose is a bit strenuous and complicated for beginners, much care should be taken in doing it. The chest should be straight, or, failing that, just a bit stooped forward. The chest should never be bent backward.

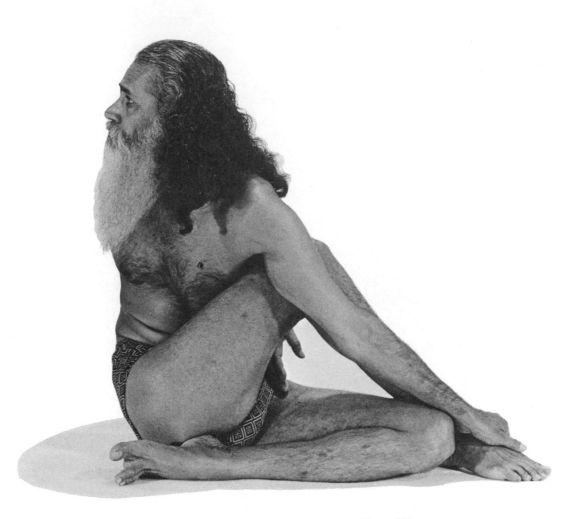

ARDDHA MATSYENDRĀSANA—*Front View*

TIME: This pose should be done once on each side, from fifteen seconds to one minute per side.

BENEFITS: This pose brings about the two side twists of the spine with maximum effectiveness. It helps in correcting enlarged and congested liver and spleen, inactive kidneys and adrenals. It aids in the cure of dyspepsia, constipation, jaundice, and obesity. It helps to tone up the sympathetic nerves and ganglia and strengthens both the deep and superficial muscles of the back.

NOTE: This pose was discovered by Yogi Matsyendra and thus bears his name. It is Arddha (half) because it is much easier to practice than the somewhat difficult full Matsyendra. For that pose, please see Cultural Poses, Section II.

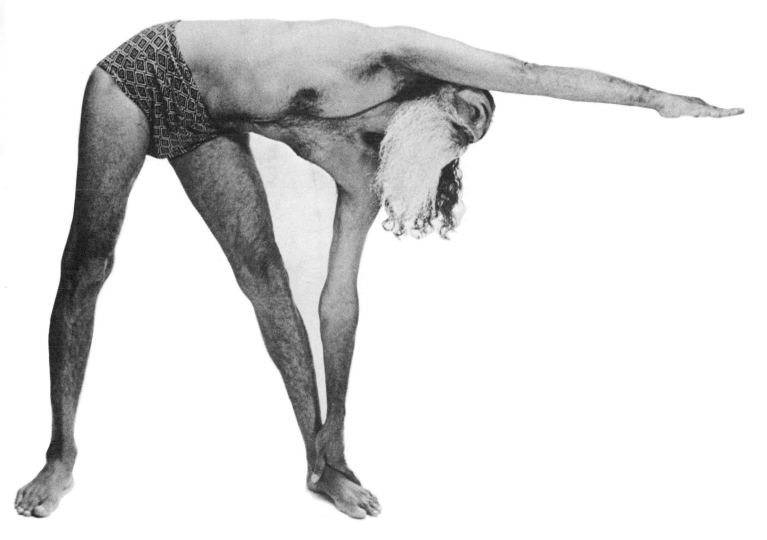

TRIKONĀSANA

15 / TRIKONĀSANA OR THE TRIANGULAR POSE

TECHNIQUE: Stand with the feet spread wide apart. Raise the arms sideways to shoulder level, with the right palm facing downward and the left palm facing up. Looking at the left palm, slowly bend the trunk of the body to the right, until the right hand reaches the right foot. Bring the left arm close to the left ear, parallel to the floor. All through this process, fix your gaze on the left palm. Then bring the trunk of the body up, raising the arms to shoulder level again, and repeat the pose on the left side. Breathe normally throughout this āsana.

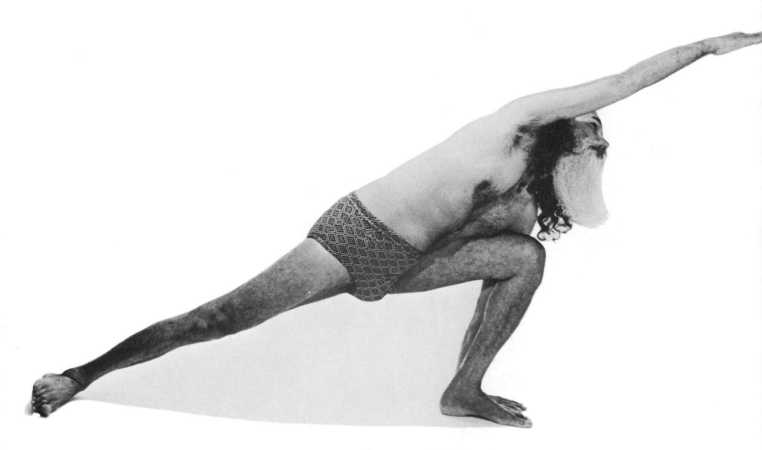

TRIKONĀSANA—*Variation*

CAUTION: Keep the knees straight throughout the pose.

TIME: Repeat three times on each side, retaining the position for ten seconds at a time. Gradually reduce this repetition and try to retain the pose just once on each side for a maximum duration of one minute per side.

BENEFITS: This pose helps to bend the spine sideways. It contracts the trunk muscles, relaxing and stretching them. Peristalsis of the bowels is increased and appetite is improved.

Variation: Stand with the feet spread wide apart. Raise the arms sideways to shoulder level. Turn the right foot and knee outward to the right. Then, bend the right knee only, and slowly go down sideways to the right, placing the right palm flat on the floor behind the right foot. The right knee should be almost against the right shoulder, and the left arm should be stretched overhead, close against the ear, with the palm facing downward. The left side, from the toes to the fingertips, should be stretched in one straight line. Repeat the pose on the left side.

TIME: Repeat three times on each side, retaining the pose for ten seconds at a time. Gradually reduce this repetition and try to retain the pose just once for a maximum duration of one minute per side.

BENEFITS: Trikonāsana Variation helps to bend the spine sideways. It contracts the trunk muscles, relaxing and stretching them. Peristalsis of the bowels is increased. Appetite is improved.

[66]

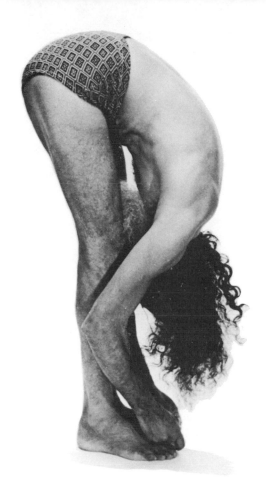

PADAHASTHĀSANA

16 / PADAHASTHĀSANA OR THE HAND-TO-FEET POSE

TECHNIQUE: Stand erect, with the feet together. Raise the arms over the head, with the palms facing forward. Exhale slowly, bend forward, and hold the toes, without bending the knees. Try to bring the face close to the knees. Breathe normally while retaining the pose, and inhale when you come up.

CAUTION: Balance yourself properly on your feet while in the pose. Do not bend the knees.

TIME: Repeat three to six times, retaining the pose for ten seconds at a time. Gradually reduce this repetition and try to retain the pose just once for a maximum duration of one minute.

BENEFITS: All the benefits of Paschimothānāsana (forward bend) are obtained through this pose. Rest is given to the heart, and the organs of the head are benefited by the great amount of blood supplied as the position of the head and heart come down below the waist.

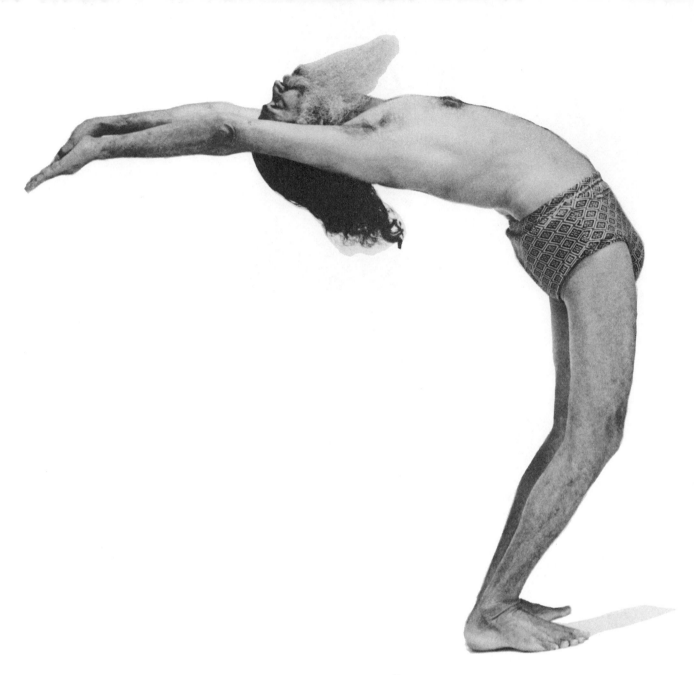

ARDDHA CHANDRĀSANA

17 / ARDDHA CHANDRĀSANA OR THE CRESCENT POSE

TECHNIQUE: Stand erect, with the feet together. Raise the hands over the head. Lock the thumbs and look at them. Stiffen the entire body from fingertips to toes. Holding the breath, bend backward to form a crescent. Hold this position as long as the breath can be comfortably retained.

CAUTION: The toes should be firm on the floor. Know your limit when bending back, for you may lose your balance if you bend beyond your capacity.

TIME: Repeat this pose three times, retaining it for two to ten seconds per time.

BENEFITS: This is an excellent anterior stretch. It is good for the entire system. The abdominal muscles are perfectly toned.

[68]

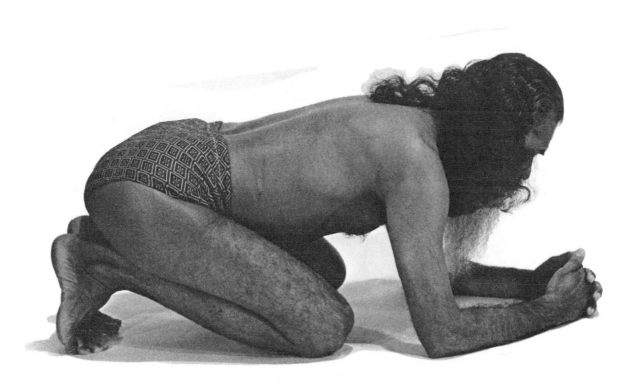

SIRSHĀSANA—*Stage I*

18 / SIRSHĀSANA OR THE HEAD STAND

TECHNIQUE (PART I):

Stage I: Kneel. Lock the fingers and create an angle on the floor with the forearms by placing them on the floor in front of you. Let the locked fingers serve as the vertex of this angle. The distance between the elbows should be a forearm's length, thus forming an equilateral triangle.

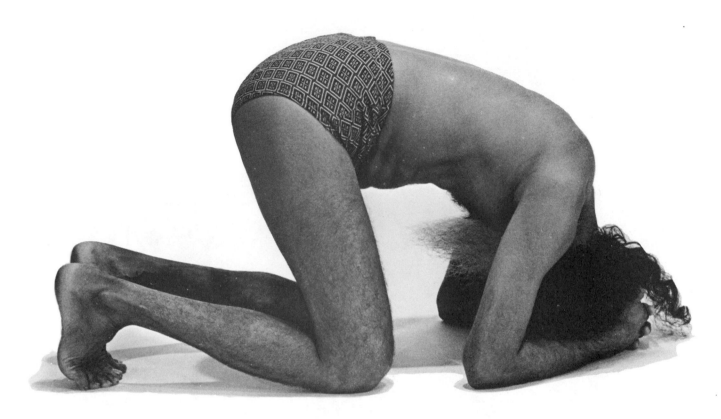

SIRSHĀSANA—*Stage II*

Stage II: Then, place the crown of the head on the floor, close to the locked fingers, so that the locked fingers can support the back of the head.

[70   ]

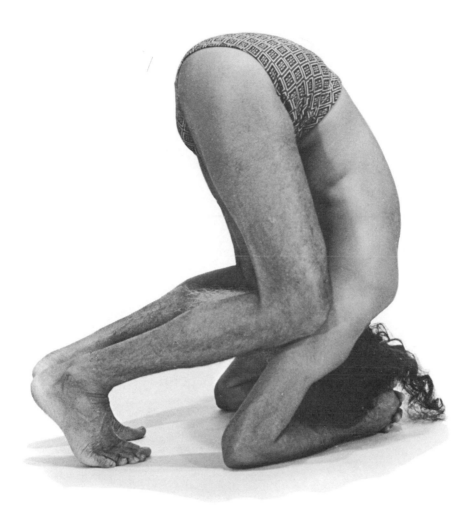

SIRSHĀSANA—*Stage III*

Stage III: Slowly lift the trunk, bringing it perpendicular to the ground. To do this, you must raise the knees and bring the toes nearer to the face. When you have raised the trunk sufficiently, you will automatically feel that the toes can be lifted slowly off the ground, without any jumping or jerking. Conversely, if the trunk is not lifted sufficiently, and if the toes are jerked up, there is every possibility of your falling backward.

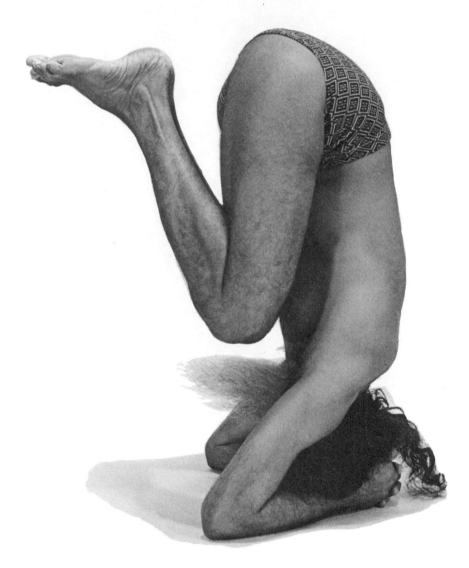

SIRSHĀSANA—*Stage IV*

TECHNIQUE (PART II):

Stage IV: After getting used to the earlier stages of Sirshāsana, slowly lift the toes and fold the legs so that the heels come closer to the buttocks, with the soles facing up.

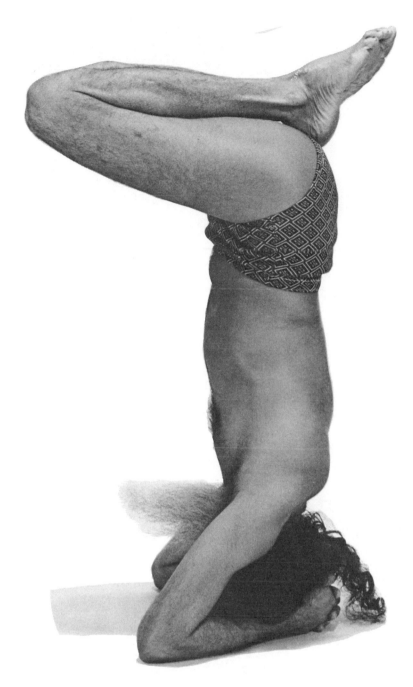

SIRSHĀSANA—*Stage V*

Stage V: Gently lift the thighs, bringing them through a horizontal position.

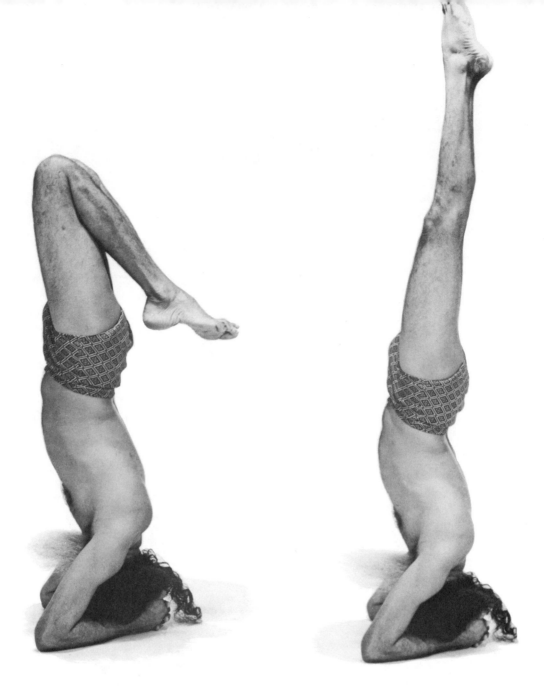

SIRSHĀSANA—*Stage VI*   SIRSHĀSANA—*Stage VII*

Stage VI: Slowly straighten the thighs in line with the trunk of the body. Keep the spine erect. Now the knees will be facing up and the legs hanging down behind the thighs.

Stage VII (Final Stage): Make sure of the balance fully before proceeding further. Little by little, unfold the legs upward to form the full pose. The weight of the body should be distributed between the head and forearms initially. Later on, the entire weight should be allowed to fall on the top of the head, with the forearms placed lightly on the floor only to maintain balance.

When coming down, reverse the order—folding the legs first, next bringing the thighs close to the chest, and then placing the knees and toes on the ground. Then, lift the head, take the forearms off the floor, and assume Vajrāsana (pelvic pose) to rest awhile and harmonize the blood circulation. Breathe normally throughout the pose.

[74   ]

CAUTION: Each stage of Sirshāsana must be practiced for several days before going on to the next stage, so that the muscles get used to the pose gradually. It is better to start practicing Sirshāsana after mastering the other poses. Never try to jerk up the legs in order to assume the pose. If there is any vomiting or nauseous feeling while doing this pose, drink half a cup of milk and begin the practice a half-hour later. Keep the mouth closed. If saliva collects, do not swallow it, but dispose of it after the pose is finished. If you feel like sneezing, coughing, or yawning while in the position, come down immediately, before doing so. Do not practice this pose if there is disturbance in the organs of the head or if headache or fever is present.

TIME: Start practice with ten seconds' duration and gradually increase the time up to ten minutes. After practicing all the poses for a good length of time, those who wish to drop the other poses may do Sirshāsana alone for from twenty-five to thirty minutes.

BENEFITS: This pose builds up a healthy brain and tones the entire nervous system. It favorably influences all the endocrine glands, particularly the pineal, pituitary, thyroid, and parathyroids. It aids in the relief of almost all nervous ailments, improves memory power, and is useful in ridding oneself of seminal weaknesses such as premature ejaculation and nocturnal emissions. It helps in the maintaining of celibacy. It helps to relieve nervous and hepatic types of asthma, as well as diseases of the lungs, digestive, and genitourinary system. Uterine and ovarian diseases are relieved. This pose benefits the body overall and helps to relieve many diseases.

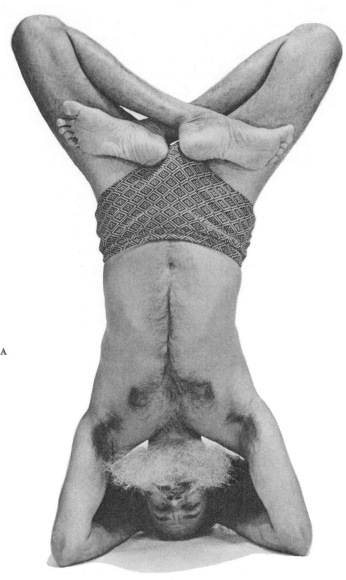

OORDHWA PADMĀSANA

19 / OORDHWA PADMĀSANA OR THE UPWARD LOTUS POSE

TECHNIQUE: Assume Sirshāsana (head stand). During the final stage, slowly fold the legs downward to form Padmāsana (lotus pose). The body should be at complete right angles to the floor, with the lotus stretched upward.

Another way of doing Oordhwa Padmāsana is to begin by sitting in Padmāsana. Place the palms, with fingers outstretched, in front of the corresponding knees, on the floor. Balance on the palms, and slide the knees over the forearms up to the elbows, bringing the head downward, with the lotus stretched up.

CAUTION: This pose calls for very strong arms and wrists.

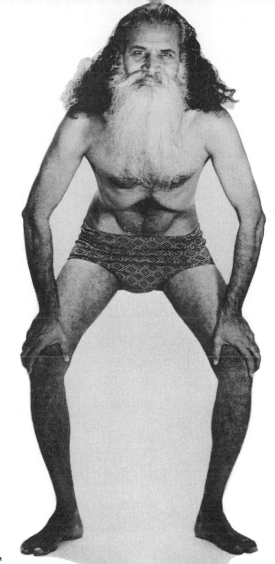

UDDHIYĀNA BANDHA

20 / UDDHIYĀNA BANDHA OR THE STOMACH LIFT

TECHNIQUE: Stand with the feet apart. Bend slightly forward, placing the hands on the corresponding knees. Empty the lungs by a deep expiration. Contract the front muscles of the abdomen and draw it in, forming a hollow. Do not inhale while this lift is being maintained. Before the breath can force its way back, release the abdomen and inhale slowly. This makes one round of Uddhiyāna. You may do this while sitting in Padmāsana, also.

CAUTION: Uddhiyāna should not be held beyond one's capacity. The moment you find that you cannot hold the breath *out* comfortably, release the muscles slowly to bring the abdomen back to the normal position. Uddhiyāna is to be avoided in cases of circulatory disturbances and serious abdominal troubles.

TIME: Repeat this pose from three to seven times, retaining the lift from five to thirty seconds each time.

BENEFITS: This is a fine exercise for the abdomen. It tones the nerves of the solar plexus. It relieves constipation, indigestion, and liver troubles; reduces abdominal fat; and strengthens flabby stomachs.

NOTE: The ancient treatises on Yoga claim that by the regular practice of Uddhiyāna, death can be conquered. This much is certain: It bestows youth and vitality. Uddhiyāna Bandha has been added to this first section on Cultural Poses because, among all the Bandhas, it is considered easy enough to be practiced by everyone.

[77]

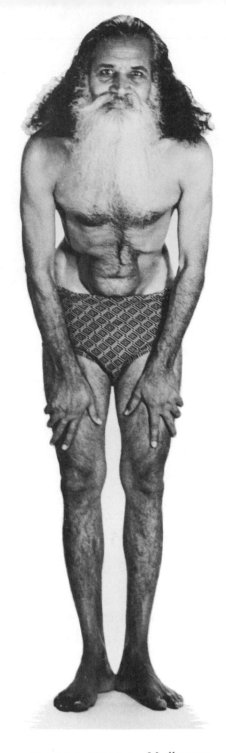

NAULI KRIYA—*Madhyama*

21 / NAULI KRIYA OR THE ISOLATION AND ROLLING OF THE ABDOMINAL RECTI

TECHNIQUE:

Madhyama or Central Nauli: Stand with the feet together. Bend forward slightly and lock the fingers, keeping them between the thighs. Rest the forearms on the thighs. Then,

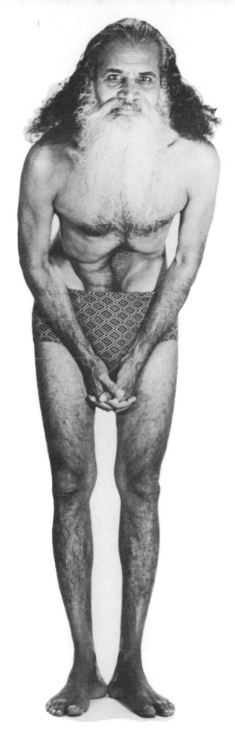

NAULI KRIYA—*Dakshina*

do Uddhiyāna Bandha (stomach lift). While maintaining Uddhiyāna, gently press the forearms against the thighs and simultaneously lift the abdominal recti forward to stand vertically in the center. Hold this position for a while, and allow the abdominal recti to go back before releasing the Uddhiyāna Bandha.

Follow the Madhyama Nauli with Dakshina Nauli and Vama Nauli.

Dakshina or Right Nauli: Do Uddhiyāna Bandha. Contracting the right rectus, isolate it to the extreme right, while the left rectus remains fully relaxed. Release.

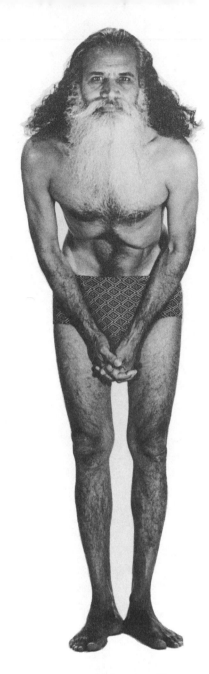

NAULI KRIYA—*Vama*

Vama or Left Nauli: Do Uddhiyāna Bandha. Contracting the left rectus, isolate it to the extreme left, while the right rectus remains fully relaxed. Release.

Nauli Proper: Do the Madhyama Nauli. Slowly roll the right rectus to the extreme right, while the left rectus is fully relaxed. Then, do Uddhiyāna Bandha and gradually bring the left rectus to the extreme left. Come back to Madhyama Nauli. This makes one round clockwise. Learn to do a few more rounds in the same way, churning without break. Reverse the above order and do the rounds counterclockwise. These rolling manipulations constitute Nauli in its strictest sense.

CAUTION: First master the Madhyama Nauli and then practice Dakshina Nauli and Vama Nauli a few times. These should also be practiced well before proceeding to the practice of rolling the recti (Nauli Proper), which is the real Nauli Kriya.

Those suffering from any type of serious abdominal illness, such as appendicitis, should not try Nauli on their own. Likewise, for sufferers of high blood pressure. Young boys and girls should not try Nauli. It should be practiced only on an empty stomach, but habitually constipated people may practice it even before having to answer the call of nature. In this case, it is best to drink one or two cups of water before practice, in order to help move the bowels.

T I M E :   Nauli should be done only to one's capacity, without any strain either on the muscles or during retention of the breath. After getting used to it, about three to seven rounds can be done, with from five to fifteen turns per round.

B E N E F I T S :   Nauli regenerates the abdominal viscera and makes the gastrointestinal or alimentary system healthy. It relieves chronic constipation and dyspepsia, as well as benefiting faulty liver, spleen, pancreas, and kidneys. Also, in women, it helps in curing almost all menstrual disorders and ovarian insufficiency.

N O T E :   Although this is a cleansing practice, it has been added to this first section on Cultural Poses because, among all the Kriyas, it is considered easy enough to be practiced by everyone.

––––––––––––––––––––––––   ⚘   ––––––––––––––––––––––––

"A short scientific survey of yogic poses drives us irresistibly to the conclusion that the advantages claimed for asanas are fully justified, and that no man wishing to develop his body, mind, and soul by taking to the practice of only one system of exercises can afford to overlook Yogic Asanas."

—SWAMI KUVALAYANANDA (*formerly* Dr. Gune)

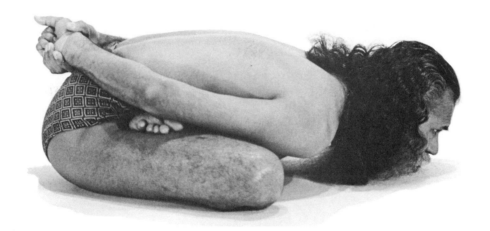

YOGA MUDRA

22 / YOGA MUDRA OR THE YOGIC SEAL

TECHNIQUE: Assume Padmāsana (lotus pose), half-lotus, or any comfortable, cross-legged position. Bring the hands in back of the body and hold the right wrist with the left hand. Slowly bend forward, as if to touch the floor with the chest. Touch the floor with the forehead first, then with the chin. Breathe normally throughout. You may exhale while bending forward, have normal breathing while retaining the āsana, and inhale while coming up. You should feel the pressure of the heels against the abdomen.
CAUTION: Those who find it difficult to reach the floor should try to bend forward only within their capacity and maintain the pose comfortably for some time. Gradually, they can try to reach the floor.

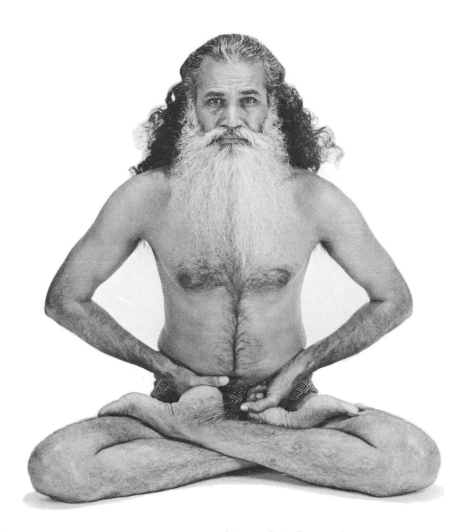

YOGA MUDRA—*Intermediate Preparation*

Yoga Mudra should be done with the āsanas, as a counterpose to Sirshāsana (head stand) and before Savāsana (corpse pose).

TIME: Repeat this pose 3 to 7 times for ten seconds at a time. Gradually reduce this repetition and try to retain the pose just once for two minutes.

BENEFITS: Yoga Mudra aids the relief of many disorders of the abdominal viscera. It tones up the nervous system, relieves constipation, and helps to overcome seminal weakness. When practiced for a fairly long time, it helps to rouse the Kundalini Sakti, or latent power, within.

NOTE: If you find this pose very easy and wish to have increased pressure at the abdomen, keep the folded fingers on the heels before you bend forward, and then do the pose. Yoga Mudra has been added to this first section on Cultural Poses because, among all the mudras, it is considered easy enough to be practiced by everyone.

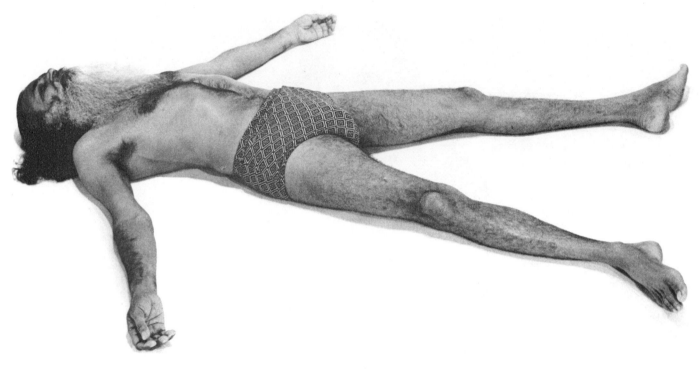

SAVĀSANA

23 / SAVĀSANA OR THE CORPSE POSE

TECHNIQUE: Lie flat on the back, placing the feet about eighteen inches apart. The hands should be slightly away from the trunk of the body, with the palms turned up. Close the eyes. Gently move all the different parts of the body to create a general condition of relaxation.

Then, start relaxing the body part by part. First think of the right leg. Inhale and slowly raise that leg about one foot above the floor. Hold it fully tensed with the breath held. After five seconds, exhale abruptly and relax the muscles of the right leg, allowing it to fall to the floor on its own, without forcing it. Shake the leg gently from right to left, relax it fully, and forget entirely about the existence of this leg. Repeat this same process with the left leg, and then with both hands, one by one.

Then, bring the mind to the muscles of the pelvis and buttocks, and to the anus. Tense them and then relax. Once again, tense and relax these muscles. Next, think of the abdominal area. Through the nose, inhale deeply, and bloat the abdomen. Hold the breath for five seconds and suddenly let the air burst out through the mouth, simultaneously feeling that all the muscles of the abdomen and diaphragm are fully relaxed. Move up to the chest and thorax region. Inhale deeply through the nose, bloating the chest. Hold the breath for five seconds, suddenly letting the air out through the mouth, simul-

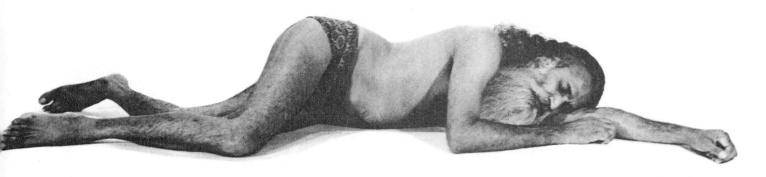

SAVĀSANA—*Variation*

taneously feeling that all the muscles of the chest and thorax are fully relaxed, as if collapsed.

Move on to the shoulders. Without moving the arms off the floor, try to make the shoulders meet in front of the trunk of the body, and drop them back to the floor, relaxed. Slowly, gently, turn the neck to the right, the left, the right, the left—back to the center— mentally relaxing the neck muscles. Coming to the facial muscles, move the jaw up and down, left and right, a few times, and relax. Squeeze the lips together in a pout, and relax. Suck in the cheek muscles, and relax. Tense the tip of the nose, and relax. Wrinkle the forehead muscles, and relax them.

Now you have relaxed all the muscles of the body. To make sure of this, allow your mind to go over the entire body, from the tip of the toes to the head, searching for any spots of tension. If you come across any tension in any part of the body, mentally concentrate upon this part and will it to relax. If you do this mentally, without moving any muscle, you will note that the part concerned obeys your command.

This is complete relaxation. Even your mind is at rest now. You may keep watching your breath, which will be flowing in and out quite freely and calmly. Watch the thoughts of your mind, without trying to take your mind anywhere. Feel as if you are the witness, not the body or the mind—the true self. Remain in this condition for some time, at least for five minutes. Do not become anxious about anything and get up abruptly. You have enough leisure at other times to allow for such thoughts. This is the time for relaxation, and only relaxation.

When you decide to wake from this so-called conscious sleep, you may do so quite slowly. Gently imagine that fresh energy is entering into each part of the body, starting from the head downward, in reverse order, to the toes. Now you may slowly sit up. I am sure you will feel quite refreshed and peaceful through the Yogic relaxation.

Variation: Lie down on the left side of the body. Stretch out the left arm and support the head with it, resting on the left cheek. Keep the right arm on the floor. The right knee should be on the floor, slightly bent and in front of the left knee. The position of the arms and legs can vary according to individual convenience. Relax the body fully and breathe gently.

BENEFITS: Lying on the left side helps the breath to flow through the right nostril, which is the sun breath.

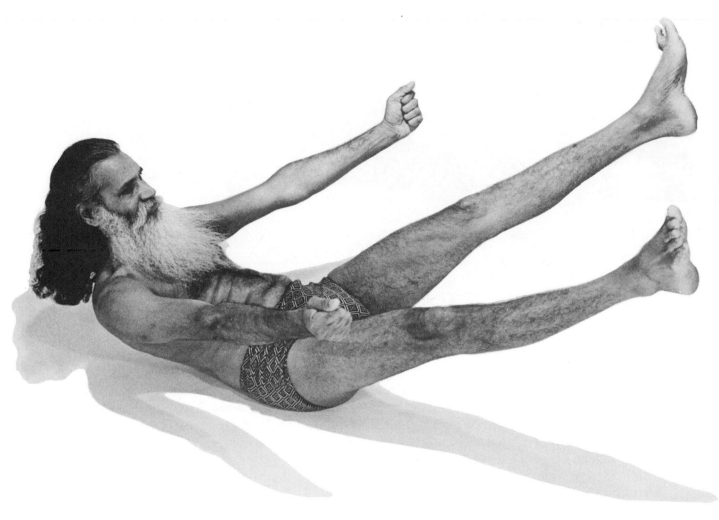

SEEGRA SAVĀSANA

24 / SEEGRA SAVĀSANA OR THE QUICK CORPSE POSE

TECHNIQUE: Lie flat on the back, placing the feet about eighteen inches apart. The hands should be slightly away from the trunk of the body, with the palms turned up.

In one motion, tighten all the muscles of the body at once, bringing the arms and legs off the floor, balancing on the buttocks. After tightening as much as possible, release all the muscles at the same time, allowing the limbs to fall to the floor on their own.

Gently shake the parts of the body from side to side—right leg, left leg, right arm, left arm. Roll the head gently from right to left.

When this has been done, follow the relaxation instructions for Savāsana.

Seegra Savāsana may be done when relaxation time is limited.

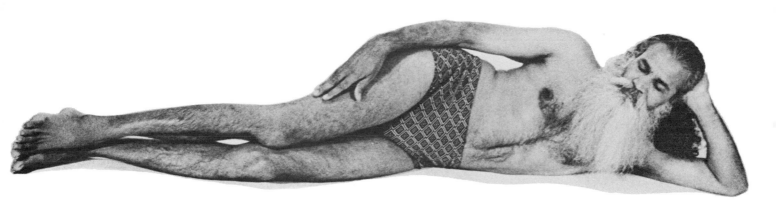

SAYANA BUDDHĀSANA

25 / SAYANA BUDDHĀSANA OR THE RECLINING BUDDHA POSE

TECHNIQUE: Lie down on the left side of the body. Fold the left arm, bringing the elbow to the floor. Stretch out the left palm and support the head with it, resting on the left cheek. Bring the right arm along the right side of the body. Bend the right leg slightly at the knee.

BENEFITS: This can be practiced whenever you want relaxation without falling asleep. It need not be practiced along with the others, but just when you want some sleepless relaxation. Lying on the left side helps the breath to flow through the right nostril, which is the sun breath.

II

As in Section I, these poses are also practiced as an aid to gaining perfect health. But in Section II are listed some of the more difficult poses and many others for those people interested in a greater number and variety of poses.

No particular order has to be followed when practicing these poses, and therefore they have been arranged alphabetically.

Time limits have not been given in this part, as it is understood that those who go to Section II will have already mastered the earlier poses and will know their capacity and time limit. Generally, each pose should be maintained for as long as is comfortable.

It is not easy to pinpoint exactly the benefits of each and every pose in this section. So instead of putting these benefits into words, we let the practitioner feel and enjoy them. Is not the proof of the pudding in the eating?

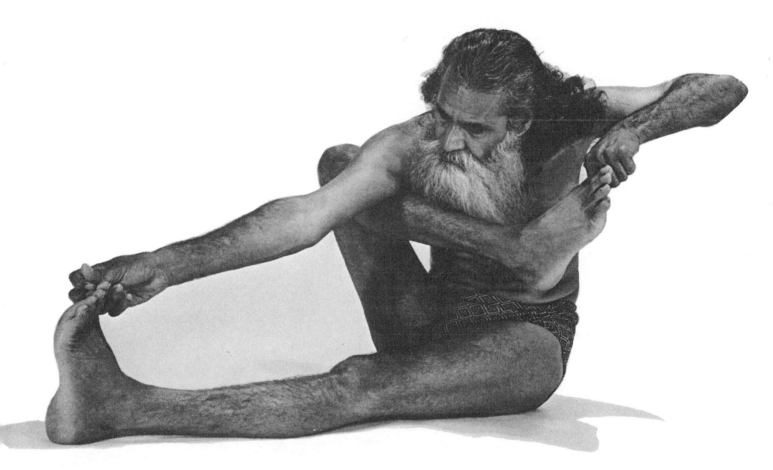

ĀKARSHNA DHANURĀSANA

1 / ĀKARSHNA DHANURĀSANA OR THE SHOOTING-BOW POSE

TECHNIQUE: Sit on the floor, with the legs stretched forward. Bend the right foot and catch hold of the right big toe with the left hand. Gently pull it back until the left hand touches the left ear. Raise the right arm over the bent leg. Bend forward, catching hold of the left big toe with the right hand.

To "shoot" the arrow, let go of the right foot and allow it to hit against the left foot. Come to the seated position again and reverse the position, bending the left foot.

[89]

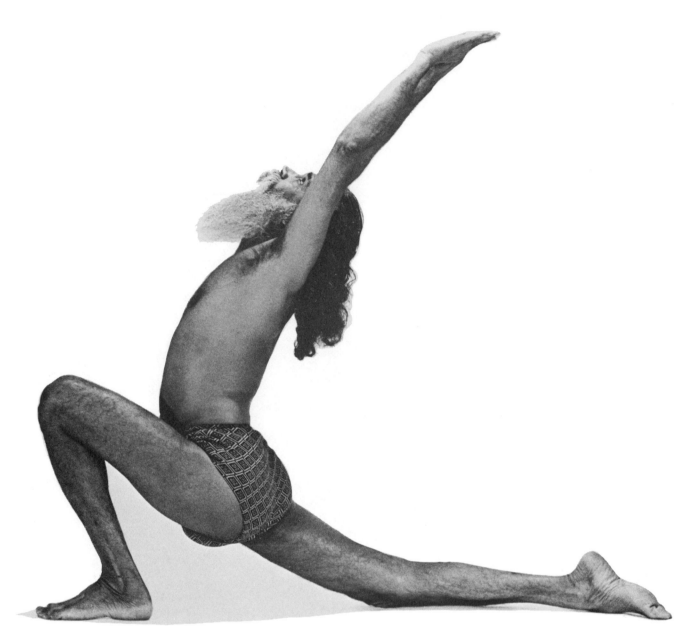

2 / ĀNJANEYĀSANA OR THE MONKEY POSE

TECHNIQUE: Stand erect. While stretching the right leg backward as far as possible, bend the left leg at the knee. Place the entire right leg on the floor. Raise the hands over the head, placing the palms against one another, and look up. Slowly bend backward, forming a "U" shape going from the hands to the leg. Come back to the standing position and reverse the pose, stretching the left leg backward.

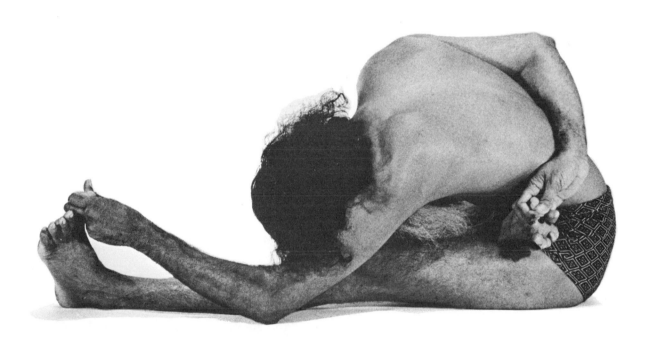

BADDHA JĀNUSHIRSHĀSANA

3 / BADDHA JĀNUSHIRSHĀSANA OR THE BOUND HEAD-TO-KNEE POSE

TECHNIQUE: Sit on the floor with the legs stretched forward. Bending the left knee, rest the left foot on the right thigh. Bring the left arm behind the back and grasp hold of the left big toe. Bend forward as much as possible, grasping the right big toe with the right hand and bringing the head to the right knee. Come up and reverse the pose, bending the right knee.

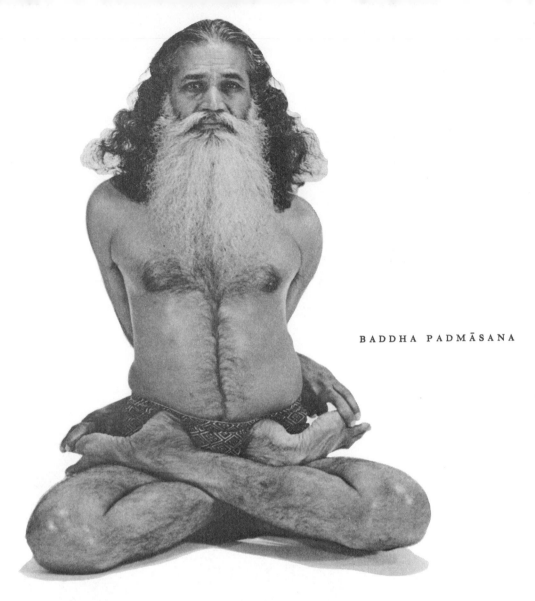

BADDHA PADMĀSANA

4 / BADDHA PADMĀSANA OR THE BOUND LOTUS POSE

TECHNIQUE: Sit on the floor and assume Padmāsana (lotus pose), pulling the feet well up on the thighs. Cross the arms behind the back, and reaching across to the opposite side with each arm, hold the toes with the hands. The right foot will then be pulled over the left thigh, held by the right arm reaching it from behind—and vice versa on the other side. While holding the feet, the big toes can be held between the thumb and the index finger. To complete this pose, press the chin against the chest and focus the gaze on the tip of the nose. If it is difficult to do the full pose, do half, and get used to it by doing it alternately on each side. This will make it easy to do the full pose later on. At the beginning of the pose, if you find it difficult, bend forward and maneuver to catch the toes and then straighten up.

BENEFITS: This pose improves general health, vigor, and vitality. It helps to relieve chronic diseases of the stomach, liver, spleen, and intestines. It helps to remove hunch. Baddha Padmāsana greatly influences the Soorya Chakra (solar plexus) and stimulates it, and thus the practitioner draws a great deal of energy in. It is also of great help in maintaining celibacy.

[92]

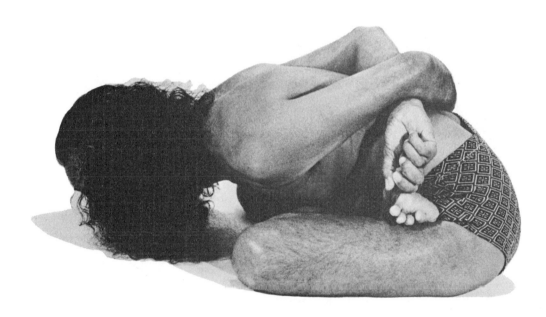

BADDHA YOGA MUDRA

5 / BADDHA YOGA MUDRA OR THE BOUND YOGIC SEAL

TECHNIQUE: Sit on the floor and assume Padmāsana (lotus pose). Pull the feet well up on the thighs. Cross the arms behind the back and hold the right big toe with the right hand, left with the left hand. Slowly bend forward and touch the floor with the forehead first and, gradually, the chin.

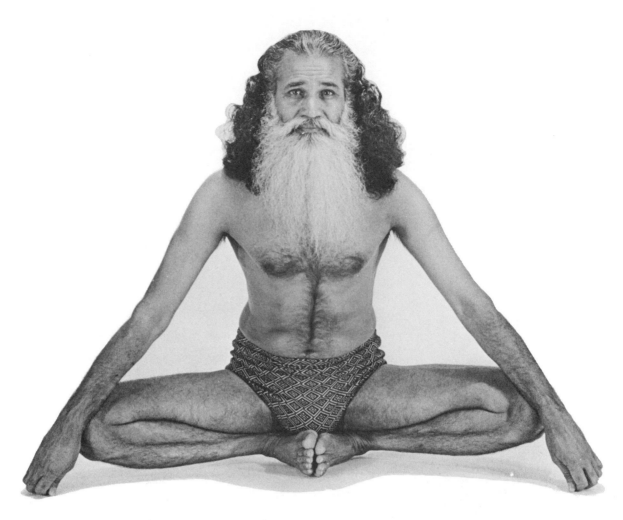

BADRĀSANA

6 / BADRĀSANA OR THE GENTLE POSE

TECHNIQUE: Sit comfortably, with the knees raised and the soles on the floor. Keep the knees apart on either side, with the soles touching each other squarely. Keeping the soles touching, draw them toward the genitals, keeping the heels under the perineum. Gently press the knees with the corresponding hands, so as to bring the knees flat to the floor. Keep the spine, neck, and head erect. Fix the gaze at the tip of the nose.

[94]

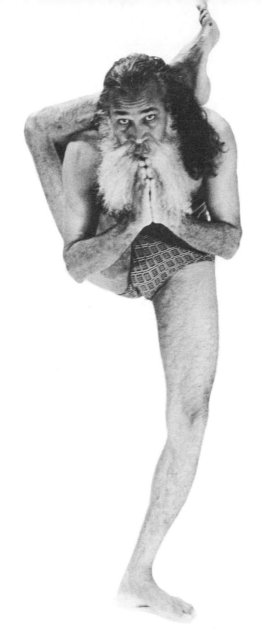

DURVĀSĀSANA

7 / DURVĀSĀSANA OR DURVASA'S POSE

TECHNIQUE: Sit on the floor with the legs stretched forward. Gently grasp the right foot, raising it over the head, and place it behind the head. Place the palms against one another in front of the chest. Now you are in Ekapādhasirshāsana (leg-to-head pose). Fold the left leg and bring the heel close to the left buttock. Press the palms against the floor for support, slowly raise the buttocks, and stand up on the left leg. Slowly come down, and reverse the pose by raising the left foot.

CAUTION: Care must be taken to maintain the balance. If there is a chance of losing the balance, immediately release the leg from the back of the neck and stand up.

NOTE: Durvasa was a sage who supposedly assumed this pose throughout his many years of penance.

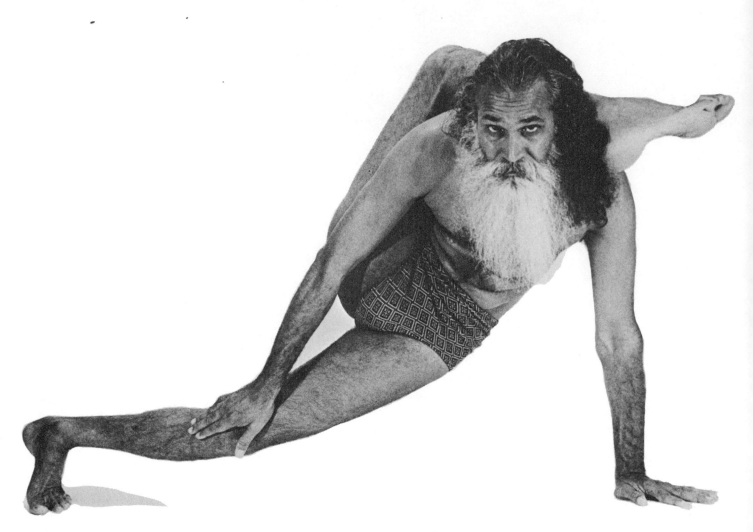

EKA PĀDA TRIKONĀSANA

8 / EKA PĀDA TRIKONĀSANA OR THE SINGLE-LEG TRIANGLE POSE

TECHNIQUE: Sit with the legs stretched forward. Gently grasp the right foot, raising it over the head, and place it behind the head. Stretch the left leg to the right side of the body. The palms should be flat on the floor on either side of the body. Putting pressure on the palms, lift up the left foot and body. Press the left toes into the floor and bring the right hand to the left knee.

[96]

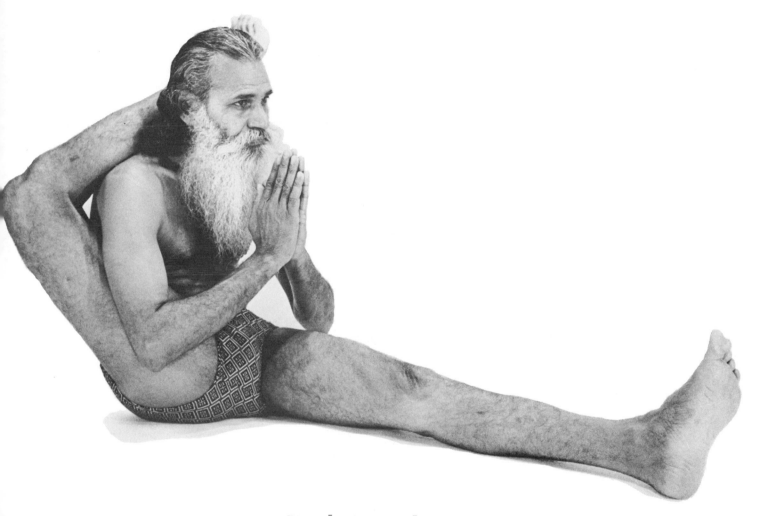

EKAPĀDHASIRSHĀSANA

9 / EKAPĀDHASIRSHĀSANA OR THE LEG-TO-HEAD POSE

TECHNIQUE: Sit with the legs stretched forward. Gently grasp the right foot, raising it over the head, and place it behind the head. Place the palms against one another in front of the chest. Come down and reverse the pose, pulling up the left leg. **Variation:** Begin the pose by lying on the floor.

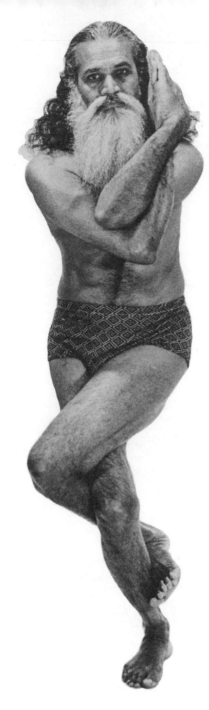

GARUDĀSANA

10 / GARUDĀSANA OR THE EAGLE POSE

TECHNIQUE: Stand up. Put all the weight on the right leg, bending it slightly at the knee. Entwine the left leg with the right. Raise the left forearm, with the palm facing the right side and the thumb against the left ear. Bring the right elbow under the left elbow. Entwine the right forearm, bringing the right palm almost against the left palm. Slowly come down and reverse the pose, putting all the weight on the left leg.

CAUTION: Take care to maintain balance.

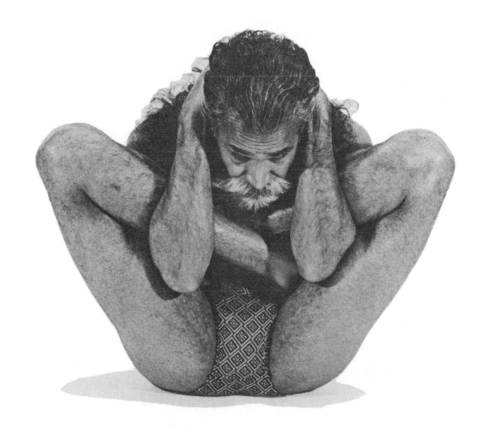

GHARBĀSANA

11 / GHARBĀSANA OR THE CHILD-IN-WOMB POSE

TECHNIQUE: Sit on the floor and assume Padmāsana (lotus pose). Bend forward, inserting the hands through the thigh and calf of the corresponding legs, as for Kukkutāsana (cock pose). Lift up the thighs and legs while maintaining Padmāsana—insert the entire length of the forearms, bringing out the elbows too. Then, raise the forearms and entwine the hands around the neck, balancing on the buttocks alone.

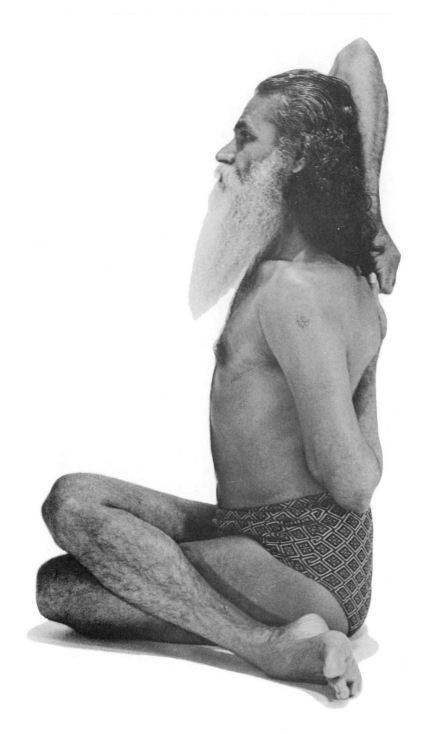

GOMUKHĀSANA—*Side View*

12 / GOMUKHĀSANA OR THE COW-FACE POSE

TECHNIQUE: Sit in Veerāsana (heroic pose), with the hands unclasped. Lift

[100]

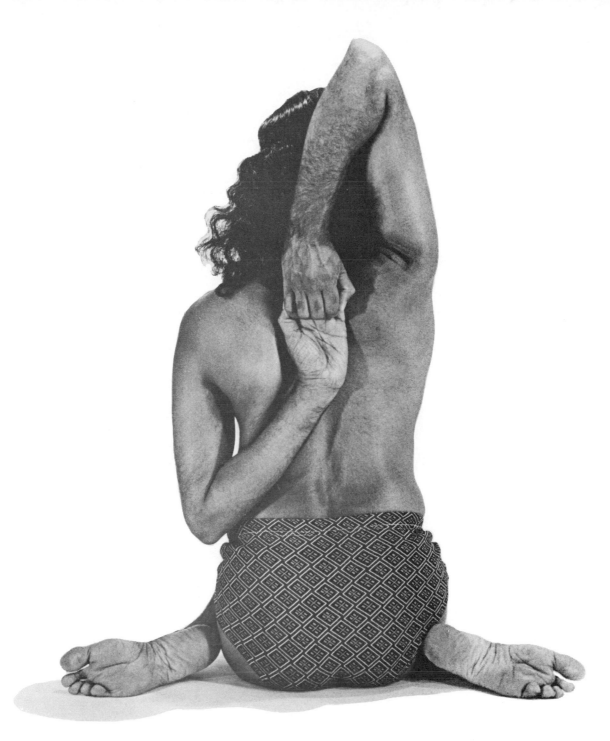

GOMUKHĀSANA—*Back View*

the right arm upward and leave the left arm down. Fold back both forearms, turning the right palm up and the left palm out. Lock the fingers at any convenient point and adjust both forearms so that they are parallel to the spine. Bring the arms down and reverse the pose, lifting the left arm upward.

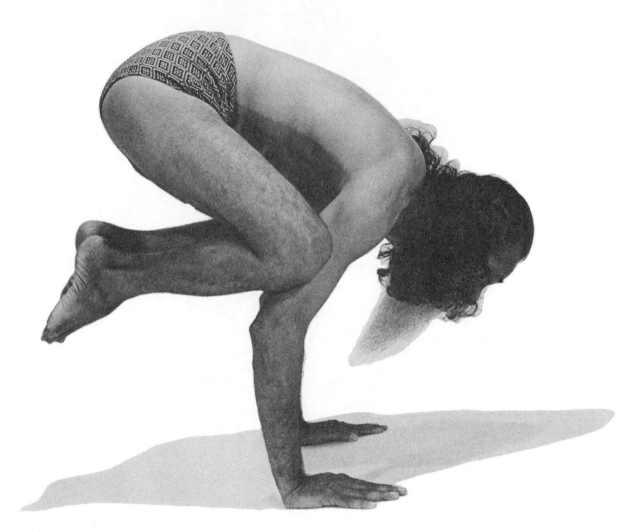

KAKĀSANA

13 / KAKĀSANA OR THE CROW POSE

TECHNIQUE: Squat on the toes with the heels raised off the floor. Keep the knees well spread apart. Place the palms on the floor, with the elbows touching the inside of the corresponding knees. Bend the arms at the elbows by bringing the face forward. Place the knees on the upper arms and, with proper balance, slowly raise the toes. The toes can be either apart or touching.

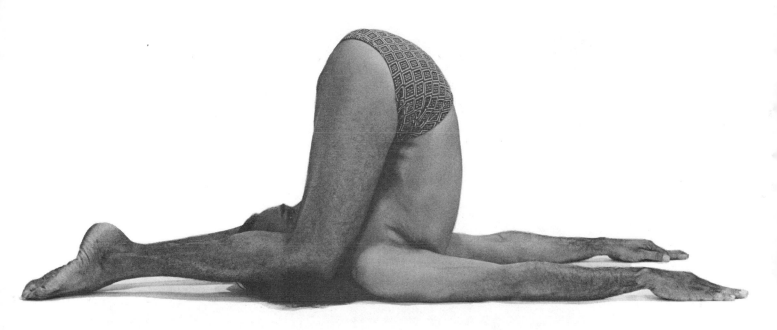

KARNAPEETĀSANA

14 / KARNAPEETĀSANA OR THE EAR-TO-KNEE POSE

TECHNIQUE: Lie flat on the back. Keep the hands alongside the body, with the palms flat on the floor. The palms should remain in that position throughout the pose. Putting pressure on the palms, raise the legs over the head and touch the floor with the toes. Walk the toes toward the head until the knees are just above the eyes. Slowly bring the knees to the sides of the corresponding ears and place the knees on the floor.

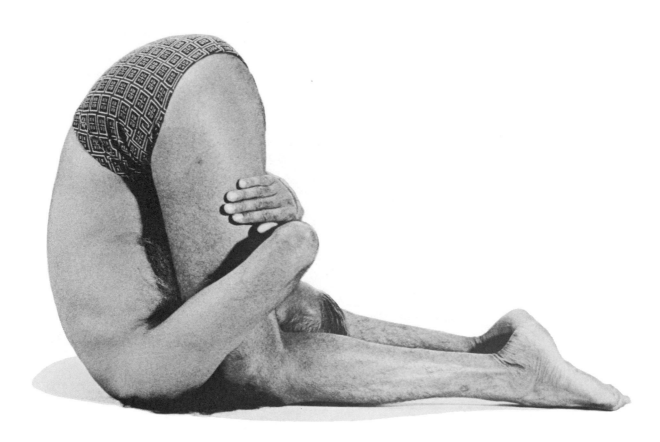

KARNAPEETĀSANA—*Variation*

Variation: Lie flat on the back. Keep the hands alongside the body, with the palms flat on the floor. Putting pressure on the palms, raise the legs over the head and touch the floor with the toes. Bend the knees and bring them to the sides of the corresponding ears. Raise the arms off the floor and bring them around the backs of the knees. Retain as long as you comfortably can.

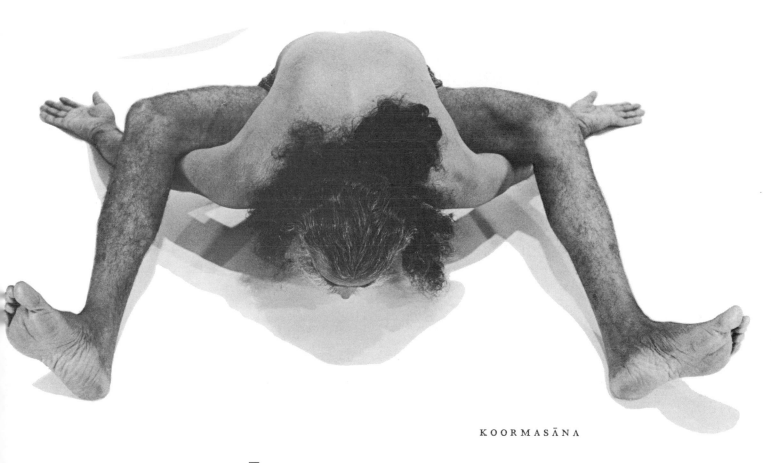

KOORMASĀNA

15 / KOORMĀSANA OR THE TORTOISE POSE

TECHNIQUE: Sit with the legs stretched forward. Spread them as far apart as they will go. Lift the knees slightly. Bend the trunk forward, bringing the head to the floor. One by one, insert the arms under the corresponding knees. Stretch the arms backward, with the palms facing up. Slowly bend forward so that the chin rests on the floor.

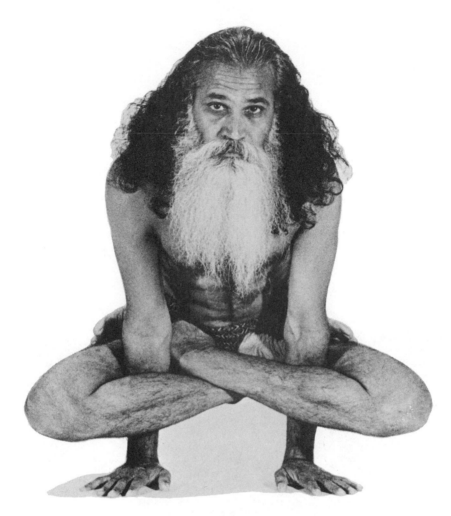

KUKKUTĀSANA

16 / KUKKUTĀSANA OR THE COCK POSE

TECHNIQUE: Sit on the floor and assume Padmāsana (lotus pose). Insert the hands through the thigh and calf of the corresponding legs. Place the palms flat on the floor. Balancing on the palms, draw up the entire lotus above the ground, sliding up as far as the elbows, so that the entire forearm is inserted through.

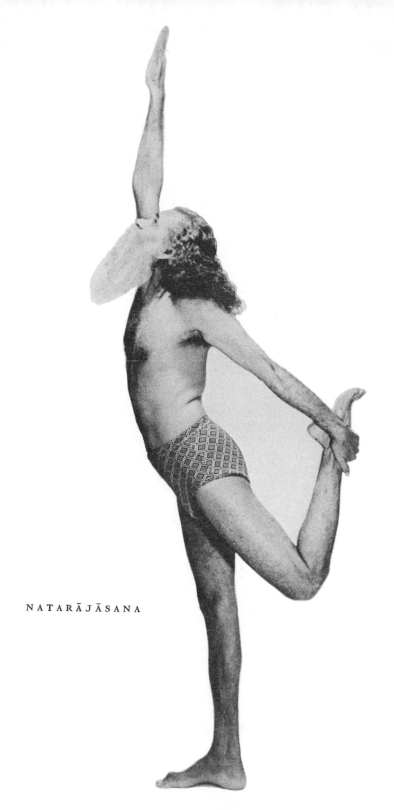

NATARĀJĀSANA

17 / NATARĀJĀSANA OR THE KING DANCER POSE

TECHNIQUE: Stand erect. Bend the right leg backward. Catch hold of the right big toe with the right arm and pull the toe toward the head. Lift the left arm straight up. Come down and reverse the pose, bending the left leg backward.

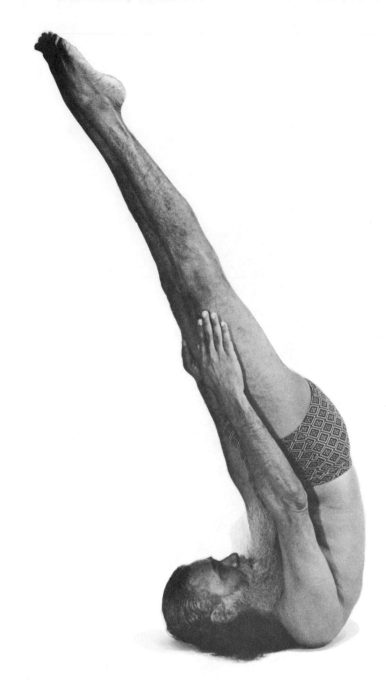

NIRĀLAMBA SARVĀNGĀSANA

18 / NIRĀLAMBA SARVĀNGĀSANA OR THE UNSUPPORTED SHOULDER STAND

TECHNIQUE: Lie flat on the back, placing the hands alongside the body. Raise the legs to a 90-degree angle. Raise the trunk to a vertical position, with the chin pressed against the chest. As you raise the trunk, simultaneously raise the forearms to support the back. Now you are in Sarvāngāsana (shoulder stand). Maintaining your balance well, slowly bring the arms up and bring the palms alongside the thighs.

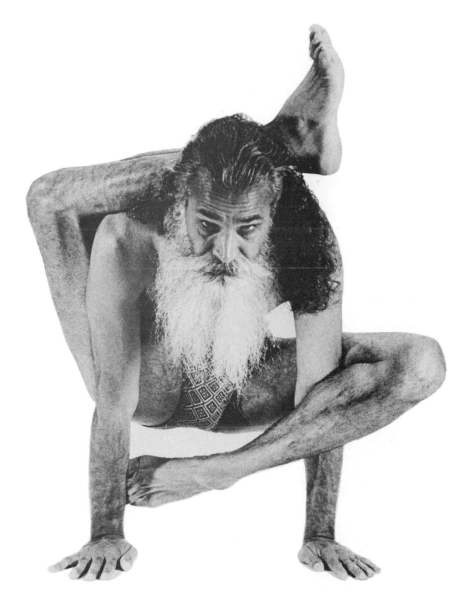

OMKĀRĀSANA

19 / OMKĀRĀSANA OR THE "OM" POSE

TECHNIQUE: Sit comfortably. Raise the entire right leg upward, bringing the right shoulder and the head forward by passing them under the right foreleg. Then, set the foreleg along the back of the shoulder with the ankle against the nape of the neck. Balance on both palms, keeping them flat on the ground in front, with the fingers pointing forward.

Suspend the body, twisting the left leg around the left forearm and letting the left foot rest against the right forearm behind the elbow. Only the palms should be on the floor.

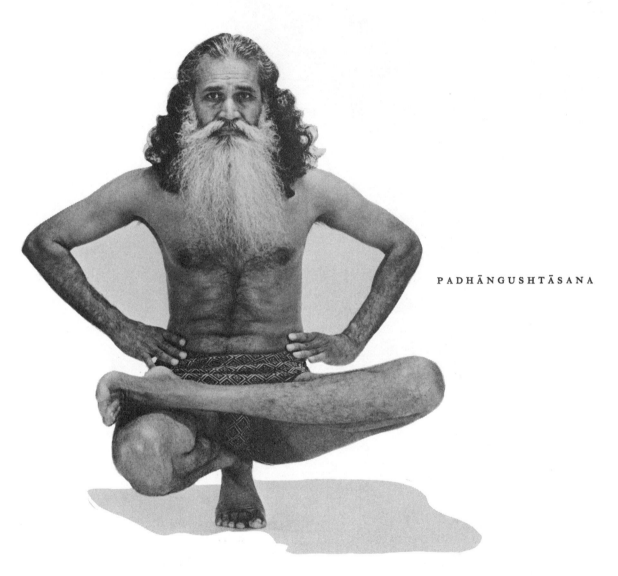

PADHĀNGUSHTĀSANA

20 / PADHĀNGUSHTĀSANA OR THE TIPTOES POSE

TECHNIQUE: Sit on your right heel with the toes on the floor. The heel should be directly in the center of the perineum. Maintaining the balance, slowly lift up the left leg and place it on the right knee. After checking the balance, slowly lift the hands, placing them on either side of the waist. Sit straight. Come down and reverse the pose, sitting on your left heel.

[110   ]

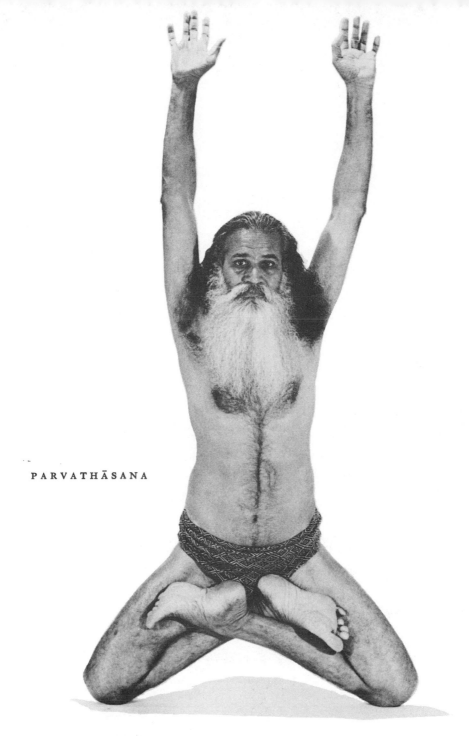

PARVATHĀSANA

21 / PARVATHĀSANA OR THE MOUNTAIN POSE

TECHNIQUE: Sit on the floor and assume Padmāsana (lotus pose). Place the palms on the floor on either side of the thighs. Slowly bend forward, raising the buttocks. When you are well balanced on the knees, move the palms flat on the floor in front of the knees. Check the balance again, straighten the trunk, and slowly raise both arms up over the head.

CAUTION: Care must be taken to maintain the balance and not fall backward or forward.

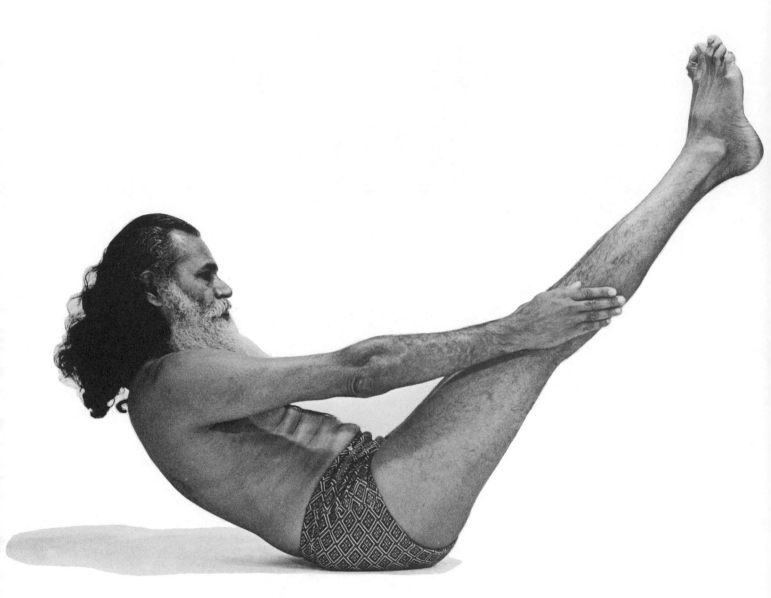

PASCHIMA NĀUĀSANA

22 / PASCHIMA NĀUĀSANA OR THE FORWARD BOAT POSE

TECHNIQUE: Lie on the back, with the legs stretched forward and the arms at the sides of the body. Raise the trunk of the body and the legs simultaneously, resting on the buttocks. Raise the arms to the same level as the knees. Keep the head between the arms and the gaze upward. Slowly come down.

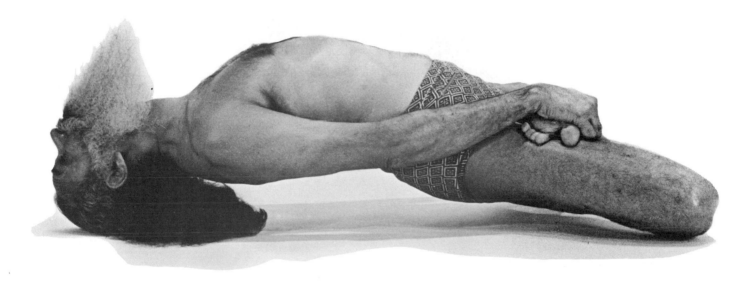

POORNA MATSYĀSANA

23 / POORNA MATSYĀSANA OR THE FULL FISH POSE

TECHNIQUE: Sit on the floor and assume Padmāsana (lotus pose). Holding on to the bottoms of the thighs, bring the elbows to the floor, one by one. Slowly bend the head backward, arching the spine and bringing the crown to the floor, as in Matsyāsana (fish pose). Bring the arms up and hold on to the right foot with the left hand, left foot with the right hand. Gradually raise the buttocks off the floor. Hold the pose as long as you comfortably can.

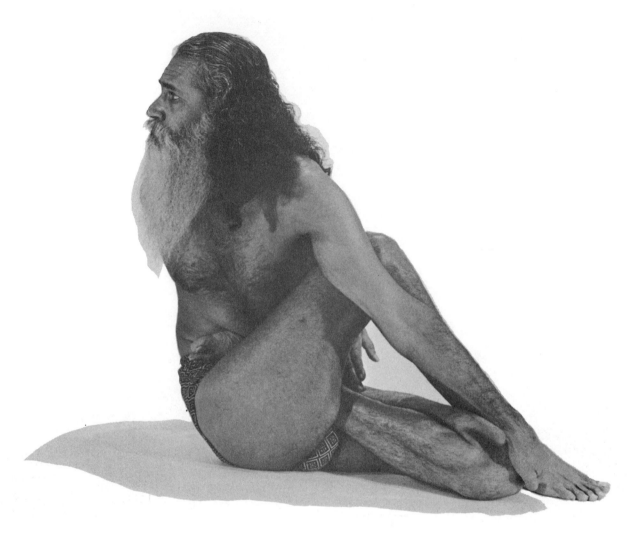

POORNA MATSYENDRĀSANA

24 / POORNA MATSYENDRĀSANA OR THE FULL SPINAL TWIST

TECHNIQUE: Sit on the floor, with the legs stretched forward. Fold back the left foreleg, placing the left foot at the base of the right thigh. The heel should be slightly below the navel, and the sole should be pressing against the abdomen.

Take the right foot over the left knee and place it flat on the floor just outside of the left knee, with the right knee close against the chest. Place hands as you would for Arddha Matsyendrāsana (half spinal twist).

The only difference in performing half spinal twist and full spinal twist is that in the half twist, the left foot is on the floor outside the right buttock, while in full spinal twist the foot is pressed between the right thigh and the abdomen.

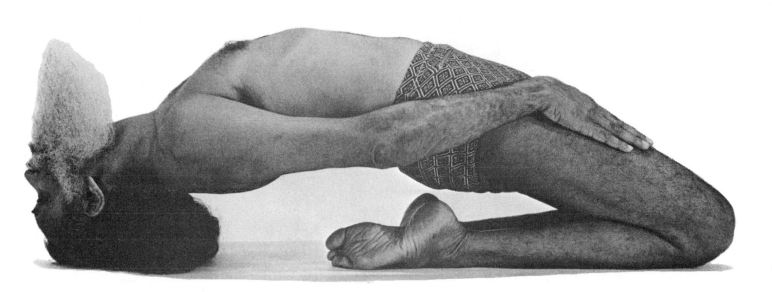

POORNA SUPTA VAJRĀSANA

25 / POORNA SUPTA VAJRĀSANA OR THE FULL BENT PELVIC POSE

TECHNIQUE: Sit on the floor. Assume Vajrāsaṅa (pelvic pose), with the palms on the thighs. Slowly bend the head backward, arching the spine and bringing the crown to the floor. This will form a curve. Raise the buttocks off the heels.

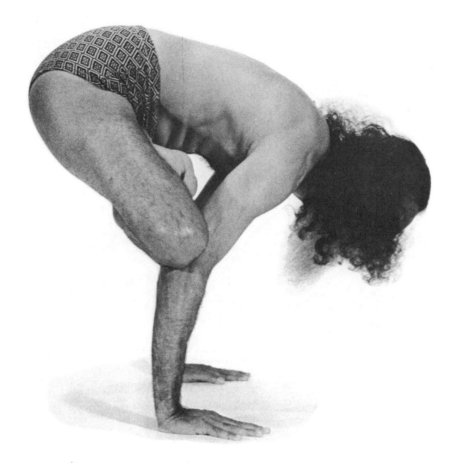

POORNA UTTHITHA PADMĀSANA

26 / POORNA UTTHITHA PADMĀSANA OR THE FULLY ELEVATED LOTUS POSE

TECHNIQUE: Sit on the floor and form Padmāsana (lotus pose). Place the palms flat on the floor, with the fingers outstretched in front of the corresponding knees. Balancing on the palms, raise the lotus up, with the knees sliding over the arms up to the elbows, and resting over them.

CAUTION: Take care not to fall on your face while elevating the lotus. If necessary, place a pillow in front of your face.

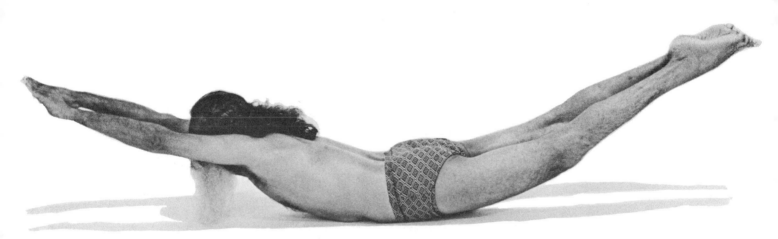

POORVA NĀUĀSANA

27 / POORVA NĀUĀSANA OR THE BACKWARD BOAT POSE

TECHNIQUE: Lie on the stomach, with the feet together and the toes stretched out. Stretch the arms over the head and lock the thumbs. Keep the head between the arms, with the arms touching the ears. Keep the gaze upward. Slowly raise the arms, head, chest, and legs off the floor, forming a curve.

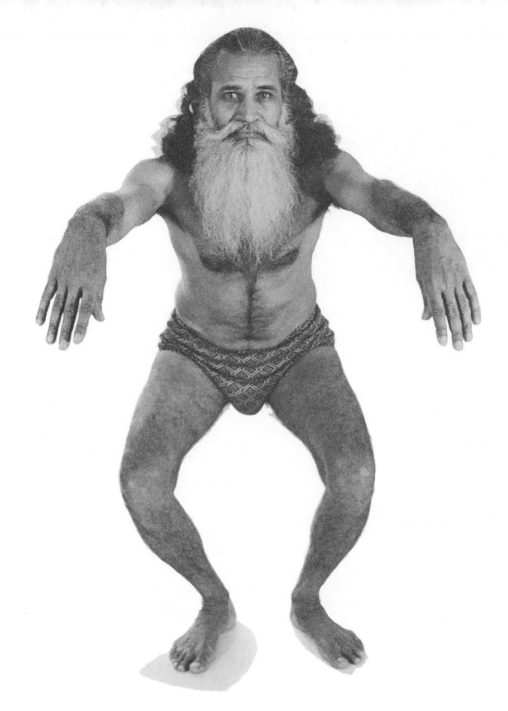

SANKATĀSANA

28 / SANKATĀSANA OR THE CHAIR POSE

TECHNIQUE: Stand up, with the feet about a foot apart. Extend the arms in front of the body, with the hands hanging loose. Bend the knees and lower the buttocks until the thighs are parallel to the floor. You should look as if you are sitting on an invisible armchair.

[118]

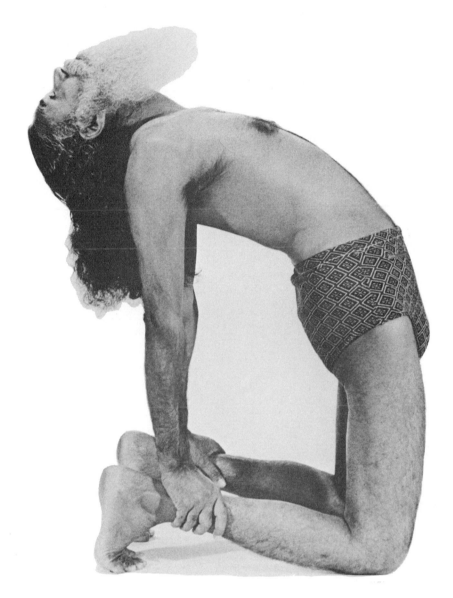

SASANGĀSANA

29 / SASANGĀSANA OR THE RABBIT POSE

TECHNIQUE: Kneel on the floor. Press thc toes into the floor. Slowly bend the head backward, looking up. One by one, grasp the ankles with the corresponding hands.

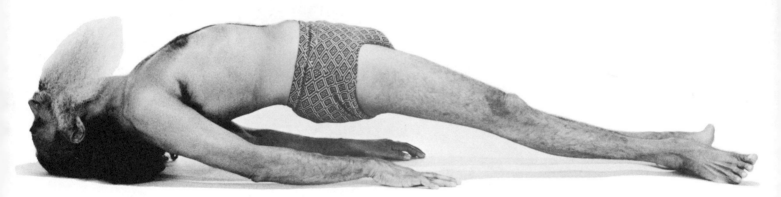

SETHU BANDHĀSANA—*Figure 1*

30 / SETHU BANDHĀSANA OR THE BRIDGE POSE

TECHNIQUE: Lie flat on the floor with the palms of the hands holding the sides of the thighs. Resting the weight on the elbows, raise the head and trunk. Bend the head

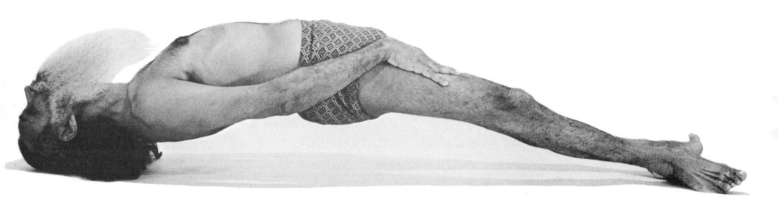

SETHU BANDHĀSANA—*Figure 2*

backward, arching the spine, and place the crown of the head on the floor. Slowly lift the buttocks off the floor, so that an arch is formed from the heels to the crown. Bring the palms to the tops of the thighs.

CAUTION: As this pose is somewhat strenuous, make sure not to strain yourself in it.

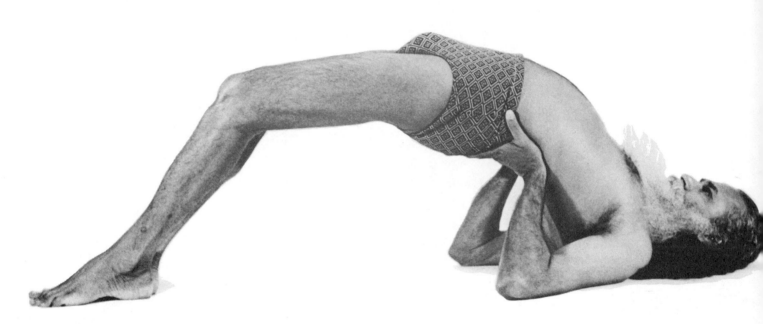

SETHU BANDHA SARVĀNGĀSANA

31 / SETHU BANDHA SARVĀNGĀSANA OR THE BRIDGE SHOULDER STAND

TECHNIQUE: Lie flat on the back, placing the hands alongside the body. Raise the legs to a 90-degree angle. Raise the trunk to a vertical position, with the chin pressed against the chest. As you raise the trunk, simultaneously raise the forearms to support the back. Now you are in Sarvāngāsana (shoulder stand). Supporting the back well, bend the knees (either one at a time or together) and bring the soles of the feet to the floor, about one foot apart. If possible, before relaxing, slowly raise the legs and trunk back to Sarvāngāsana and then come down.

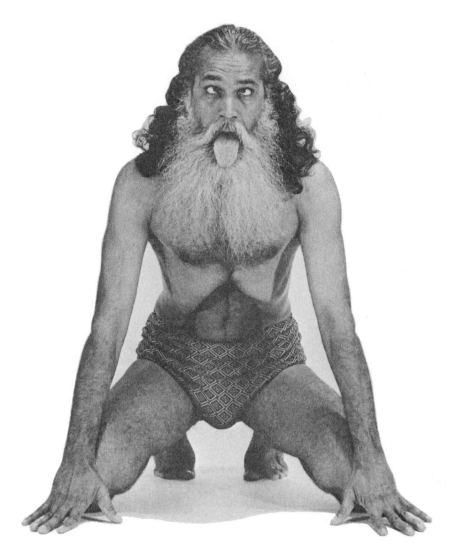

SIMHĀSANA

32 / SIMHĀSANA OR THE LION POSE

TECHNIQUE: Kneel down, keeping the toes together and placing the knees about one foot apart. Sit back on the raised heels, so that only the toes and knees touch the floor. Then, lean slightly forward, placing the palms on the corresponding knees, with the arms and fingers outstretched. Exhale and draw in the stomach muscles as for Uddhiyāna Bandha (stomach lift). Let the tongue hang out as far as possible, and focus both eyes on a spot between the eyebrows. Tense the whole body. Inhale; straighten body.

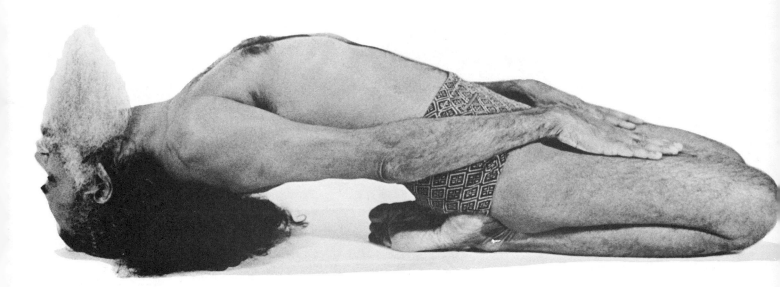

SUPTA VAJRĀSANA

33 / SUPTA VAJRĀSANA OR THE BENT PELVIC POSE

TECHNIQUE: Sit on the floor. Assume Vajrāsana (pelvic pose), with the palms on the thighs. Slowly bend the head backward, arching the spine and bringing the crown to the floor. This will form a curve.

NOTE: This is actually Matsyāsana (fish pose) done with the feet in Vajrāsana instead of straight out or in Padmāsana (lotus pose).

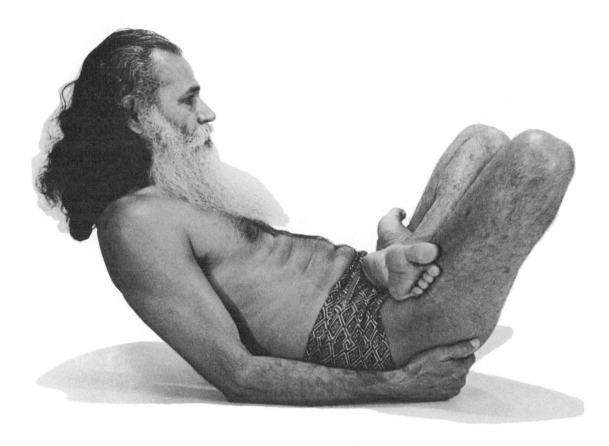

TOLANGULĀSANA

34 / TOLANGULĀSANA OR THE SCALE POSE

TECHNIQUE: Lie on the back and assume Padmāsama (lotus pose). Lift the entire lotus and buttocks and place your wrists with closed fists underneath the buttocks, facing down. Then, raise the trunk also. Balance in this position.

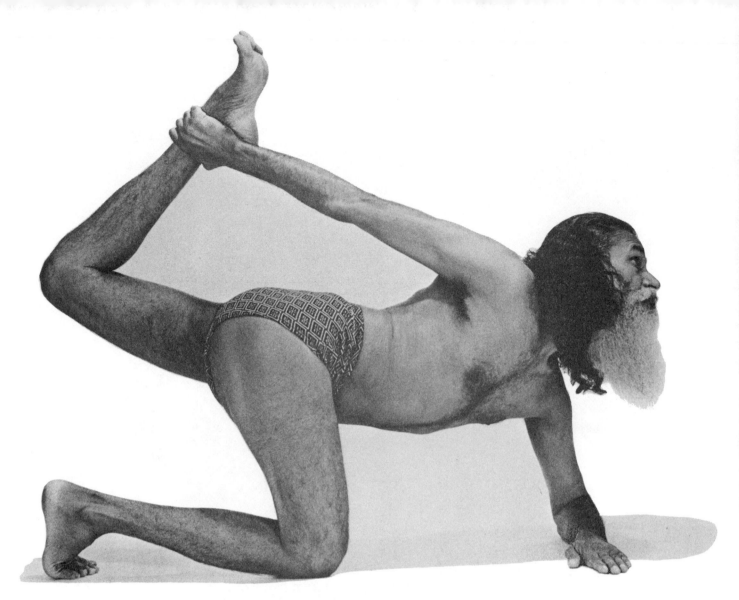

UTTHITHA DHANURĀSANA

35 / UTTHITHA DHANURĀSANA OR THE RAISED-BOW POSE

TECHNIQUE: Position yourself on the floor "on all fours." Place the left fore-arm on the floor, parallel to and under the shoulder line, with the left palm flat on the floor. Place the right knee on the floor. The body should rest on the right leg and left arm. Grasp the left ankle with the right hand. Distribute the weight of the body on the left arm and right leg, particularly on the left elbow. Relax the back and gently raise the left foot, without losing your grip. Look up at the ceiling. Slowly come down to the floor and reverse the position, grasping the right ankle with the left hand.
CAUTION: Avoid grasping the right ankle with the right hand or the left ankle with the left hand.
NOTE: This pose can be practiced by women during menstruation and throughout pregnancy. It helps to alleviate tension in the back muscles.

[126]

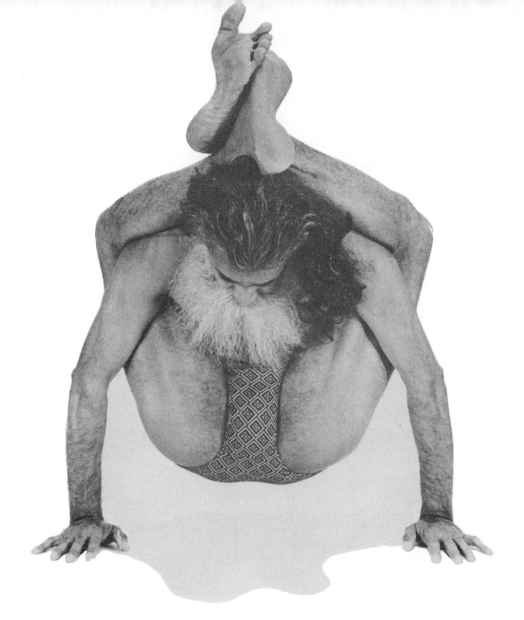

UTTHITHA KOORMĀSANA

36 / UTTHITHA KOORMĀSANA OR THE LIFTED TORTOISE POSE

TECHNIQUE: Sit with the legs stretched forward. Bend the knees toward the trunk. Bend the trunk slightly. Grasp hold of the right foot and slowly bring the right leg behind the head. Maintaining the balance well, grasp hold of the left foot, bringing the left leg behind the head. Interlock the feet at the ankles. Place the palms flat on the floor on either side of the buttocks. Putting the weight on the hands, lift the trunk off the floor.

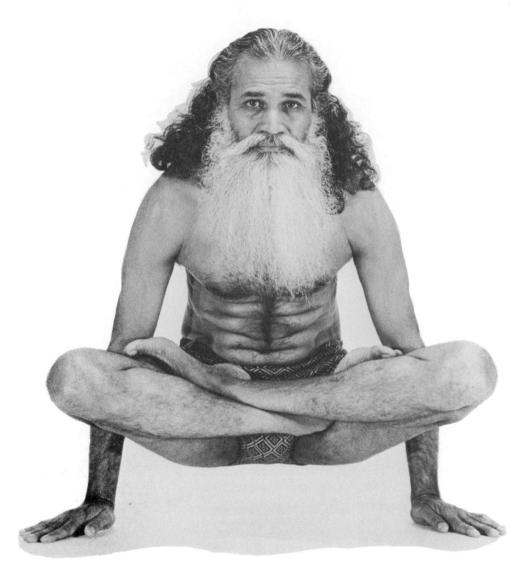

UTTHITHA PADMĀSANA

37 / UTTHITHA PADMĀSANA OR THE LIFTED LOTUS POSE

TECHNIQUE: Sit on the floor and assume Padmāsana (lotus pose). Place the palms flat on the floor on the outside of the corresponding thighs. Putting the weight on the palms, lift the trunk and the lotus-formed legs off the floor.

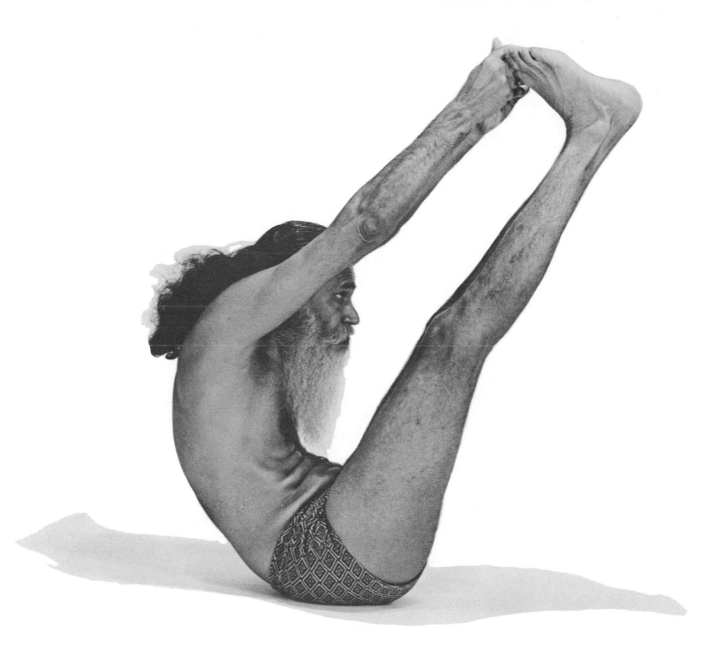

UTTHITHA PASCHIMOTHĀNĀSANA

38 / UTTHITHA PASCHIMOTHĀNĀSANA OR THE LIFTED FORWARD-BENDING POSE

TECHNIQUE: Lie on the back with the legs stretched forward and the arms at the sides of the body. Raise the trunk and the legs simultaneously, resting on the buttocks. Slowly raise the arms and grasp hold of the toes. Balance on the buttocks well. Keep the head between the arms and the gaze upward.

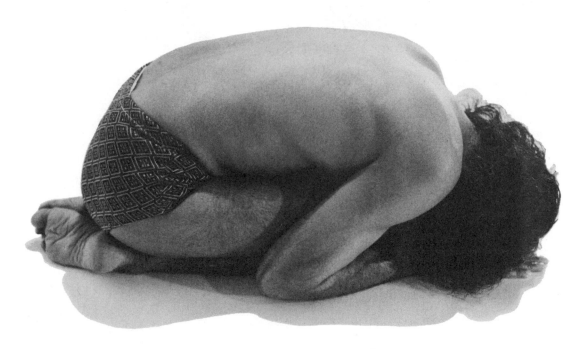

VAJRĀSANA—*Variation I*

39 / VAJRĀSANA OR THE PELVIC POSE

TECHNIQUE:

Variation I: Sit on the floor and assume Vajrāsana (pelvic pose). Bend the trunk forward, bringing the forehead to the floor. The palms should be flat on the floor, under the face and knees. Make sure the buttocks and heels are touching.

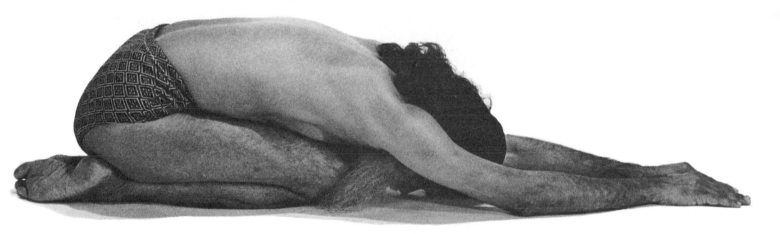

VAJRĀSANA—*Variation II*

Variation II: Assume the above position and stretch the arms over the head, with the palms touching the floor.

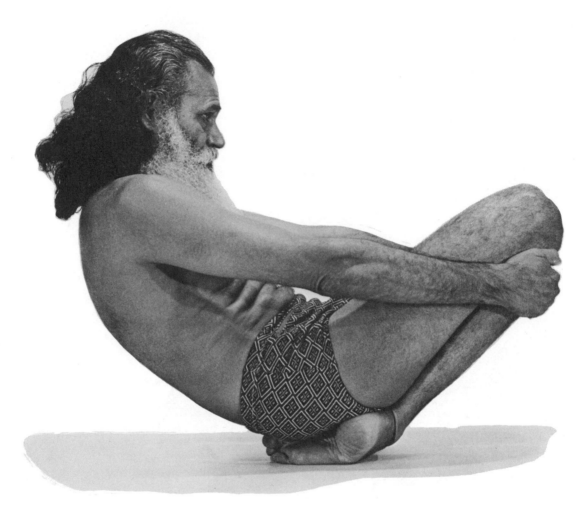

VAJRA TOLANGULĀSANA

40 / VAJRA TOLANGULĀSANA OR THE PELVIC SCALE POSE

TECHNIQUE: Sit on the floor and assume Vajrāsana (pelvic pose). Bring the hands under the knees and gently lift them, balancing on the feet.

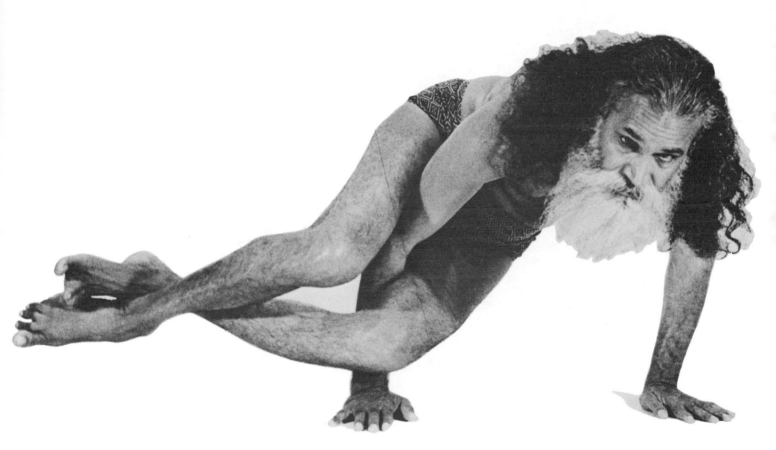

VAKRĀSANA

41 / VAKRĀSANA OR THE CROOKED POSE

TECHNIQUE: Sit on the floor and assume Vajrāsana (pelvic pose). Place the palms in front of the knees and spread them about two feet apart. Slowly bend the elbows and bring the right thigh onto the left elbow. Keep the right leg straight. Lift the left leg, bringing it in front of the right arm. Entwine the right leg with the left. The right arm should be between the thighs, with the palm flat on the floor. The balance will be on the palms, and the legs will be above the floor. Slowly come down and reverse the pose, bringing the left thigh onto the right elbow.

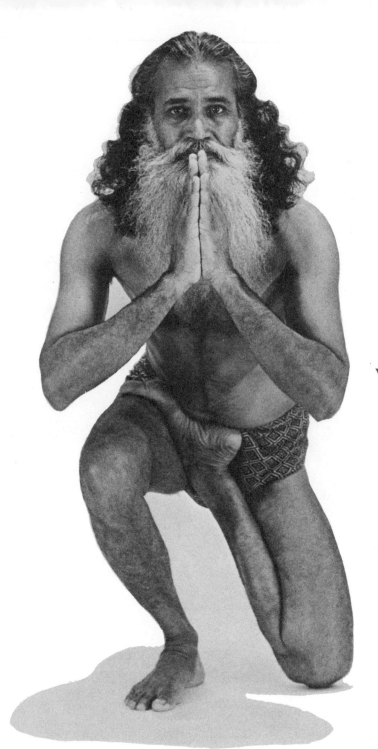

VĀTHAYĀNĀSANA

42 / VĀTHAYĀNĀSANA OR THE FOOT-AND-KNEE POSE

TECHNIQUE: Stand erect. Bring the left foot up onto the right thigh joint. Fold the arms, placing the palms against one another close to the chest. Slowly bend the right leg until the left knee touches the floor. Come down and reverse the pose, bringing the right foot up.

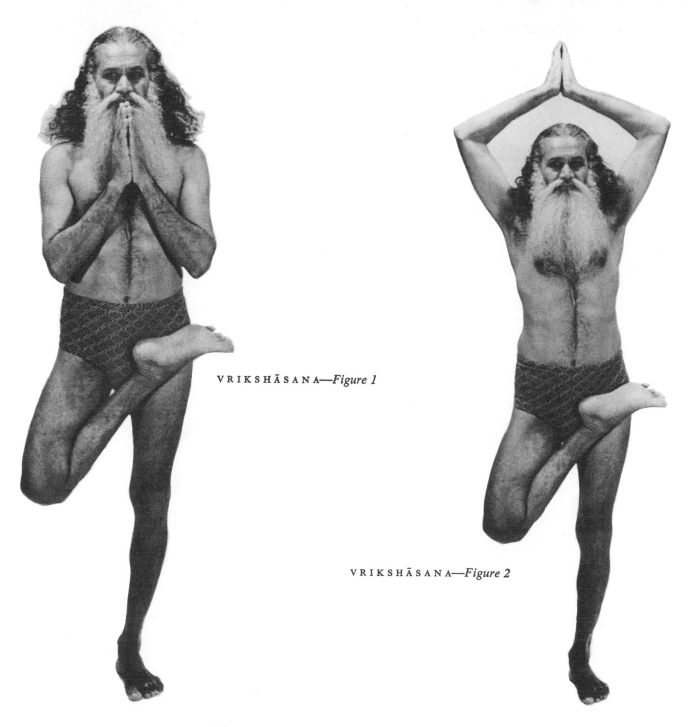

VRIKSHĀSANA—*Figure 1*

VRIKSHĀSANA—*Figure 2*

43 / VRIKSHĀSANA OR THE TREE POSE

TECHNIQUE: Stand up. Put all the weight on the right leg and fold up the left leg, fitting the left foot over the upper part of the right thigh. Bring the palms together close to the face, or raise them over the head. Slowly come down and reverse the position, putting all the weight onto the left leg.

Variation: Stand up. Put all the weight on the right leg, folding the left leg, so that the left sole is along the inner part of the right thigh and the left heel touches the genitals. Proceed as in original tree pose.

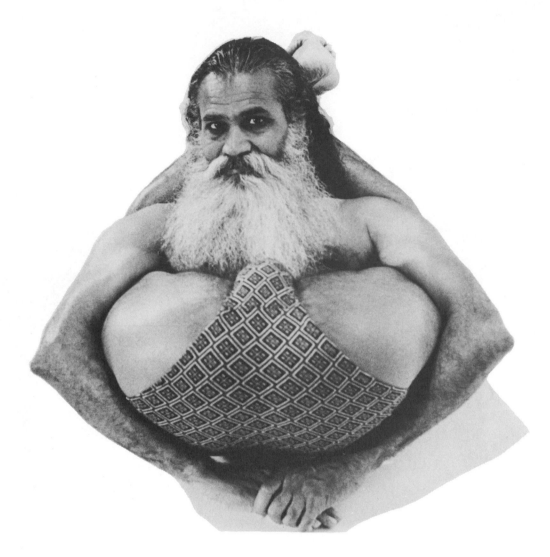

YOGA NIDRĀSANA

44 / YOGA NIDRĀSANA OR THE YOGIC SLEEP

TECHNIQUE: Lie flat on the back. Raise the right leg up with both hands, bringing the right shoulder and the head forward. Place the right ankle against the nape

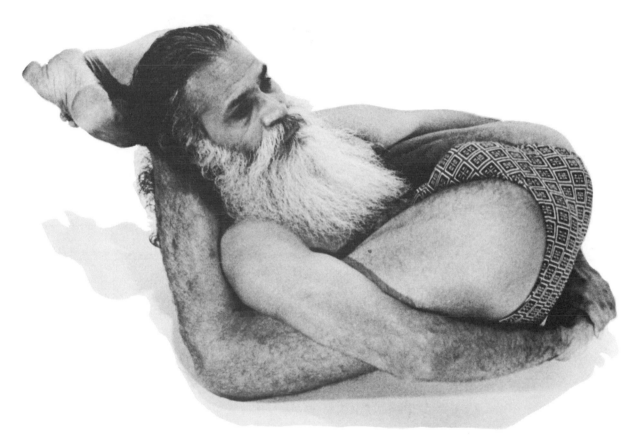

YOGA NIDRĀSANA

of the neck, as is done for Omkārāsana (om pose). Do the same thing with the left leg, so that the feet cross each other at the ankles. Circle the arms downward, to meet at a point beneath the buttocks. Your neck will then be resting on the crossed ankles. Breathe normally, stay in this pose as long as you can comfortably do so, and then slowly undo the pose, reversing the order.

PART FIVE

PRĀNĀYĀMĀS

"**P**rānāyāma" means control of prana. "Prana" is our very life, the absolute force which is present everywhere and which causes even the most subtle movements—for example, mental modifications. We can live for many weeks without food, days without water, minutes without air, but not even for a fraction of a second without prana.

By the regular practice of prānāyāma, we are able not only to control and direct the prana that functions within us, but to control and direct the universal prana as well. This is done through our thought—the agent which directs the prana.

The sage Bhagavan Pathanjali, Father of Yoga Philosophy, said, "Control of thought forms is Yoga." Those who have control over their inner prana can store it in their system and use it to heal others by mentally transmitting a portion of their supply to those in need. By their touch alone, these people can cure many ailments. Such people, however, must beware not to use this power just for the sake of exhibitions, or such egoistic involvements will certainly cause their downfall from the path to Self-Realization.

Yoga does not strive for the attainment of psychic powers, although these powers are a by-product of Yoga. Rather, the object of Yoga is perfect health, happiness, and peace of mind—and not possession of these sometime after this life, but right here and now. Another object of Yoga is to give perfect health, happiness, and peace of mind to our fellow beings.

The breath is the external manifestation of prana. We breathe about fifteen times a minute. In a normal breath, we take in and give out about one pint of air. If we use a little force, and inhale deeply, we can take in another three pints of air. In addition to our normal exhalation, if we use force to exhale further, we can exhale another three pints of supplementary air. However, even after this deep exhalation, there will still remain another three pints of residual air. Using some simple mathematics, you can figure out how much air you can inhale after a forcible, deep exhalation:

Normal Air	1 Pint
Supplementary Air	3 Pints
Complementary Air	3 Pints
Total	7 Pints

If you add to this the three pints of residual air, you get ten pints, which is the lung capacity. So, you can imagine the amount of extra oxygen and prana you can get by deep breathing—about seven times the normal quantity. This means supercharging the blood with oxygen and prana, which, in turn, brings extra life. The richness of the blood is the basis of the entire body's health, and the blood can be called rich only if it contains the necessary amount of oxygen and elements of nutrition. These are the outcome of proper respiratory and digestive functions, and the practice of prānāyāma helps bring this about.

The main product of prānāyāma is, in Pathanjali's words, "Thadhā Ksheeyatē Praka Shavaranam"—"By prānāyāma the covering of the chita [the mental stuff] is removed," and the mind becomes fit for dhārana (concentration). Therefore, prānāyāma is worth practicing for the sake of both physical and mental health.

Posture for Prānāyāma: Any sitting posture may be used for performing prānāyāma, as long as the spine is erect and the hands rest on the knees. However, it would be more profitable if any one of the meditation postures were assumed. The main meditative poses are Siddhāsana (accomplished pose), Padmāsana (lotus pose) and Swastikāsana (favorable nose). The practice of Ujjayi prānāyāma, though, may be done even while standing or walking.

Time Limit for Prānāyāma: Time limits are not given for all of the exercises in this section. In those where a limit is not given, the practitioner should use his own discretion and practice that exercise according to his own capacity.

A Note of Warning: Prānāyāma is a very powerful practice, which can bring certain extraordinary powers. Those who do not adhere to the rules of Yama and Niyama, the Yogic "Commandments," and who do not possess good control over the mischievous mind, might be tempted to misuse these powers. Therefore, prānāyāma should be approached carefully. Even while practicing, you should feel you are playing with a serpent.

Because you are dealing with such delicate organs as the lungs, the heart, and the nerve centers, you should take great care not to strain any part of the system by overdoing your practice.

This note should not scare anyone, however, because when prānāyāma is practiced faithfully, with full attention toward all the instructions given, you need not fear any harm. On the other hand, you will be bestowed with perfect health, dynamic strength, and supreme peace.

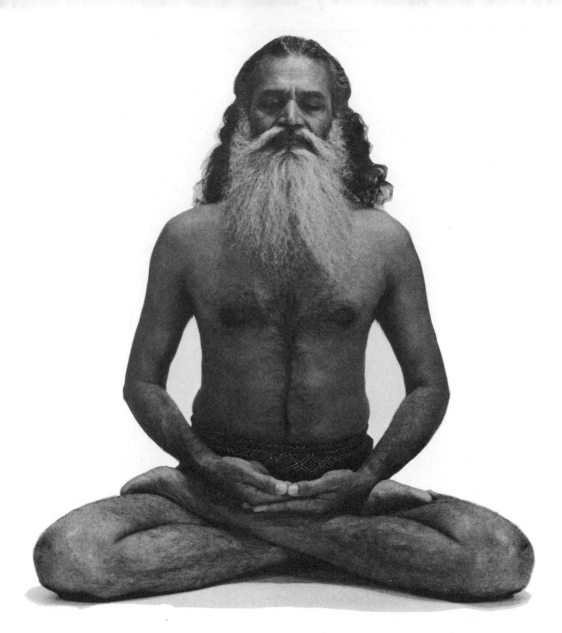

DEERGHA SWĀSAM

1 / DEERGHA SWĀSAM OR THE DEEP BREATHING

TECHNIQUE: Assume a meditative pose. Exhale slowly. Then inhale slowly. As you do so, expand the stomach and then the chest well to allow the maximum amount of air in. You may raise the collarbones also. The abdominal muscles will automatically slightly contract as the chest becomes full. Soon after, without holding the breath, exhale slowly. First drop the collarbones; then contract the chest and then the stomach, one section flowing into the other. In both inhalation and exhalation, the breath should be one continuous flow. Repeat this breathing, slowly and steadily. This method fills the lungs to capacity and empties them thoroughly.

HINT: Every inhalation should begin from the stomach, and every exhalation from the top of the lungs.

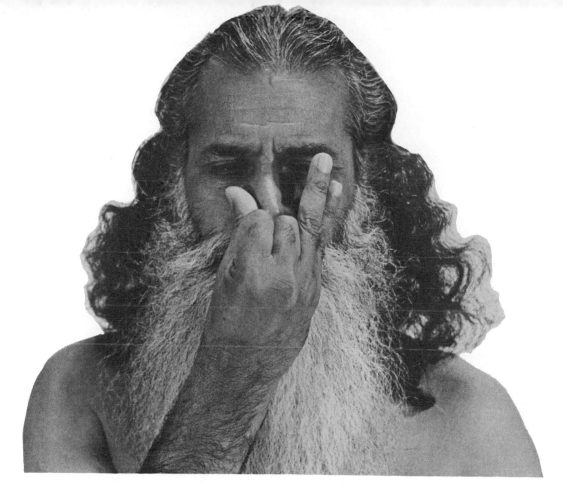

NĀDI SUDDHI—*Right Side*

2 / NĀDI SUDDHI OR THE NERVE PURIFICATION

TECHNIQUE:

Stage I: Sit in a meditative pose. Calm the mind. Watch the breath for a minute, with full concentration. Then, assume the Vishnu Mudra (please see p. 158) and close the right nostril with the thumb. Exhale slowly through the left nostril as much air as possible without any strain. At the end of this exhalation (Rechaka), slowly—without any sudden jerk—start inhaling (Puraka) through the same, left nostril. Take a slow, steady, long, deep breath. During Puraka, expand the stomach and then the abdominal muscles will automatically slightly contract as the chest becomes full, thereby allowing the maximum amount of air to go in.

At the end, gently change nostrils by closing the left nostril with the ring finger and pinky, releasing the thumb. Start the exhalation slowly and steadily—without any sudden jerk—till you feel that the lungs are almost empty. During Rechaka, slowly allow the chest to shrink, while having good control over the lungs. After the chest shrinks, slightly contract the abdomen to expel the maximum amount of air.

Now, again start the inhalation without jerking, allowing the air to flow in slowly and steadily. Again change the nostrils, and repeat this process as many times as you can comfortably and conveniently do so. Have an account of the number of inhalations and exhalations you are able to do in one round, without straining. Finishing this, take a few normal breaths, which should give you a sufficient rest and which should prepare

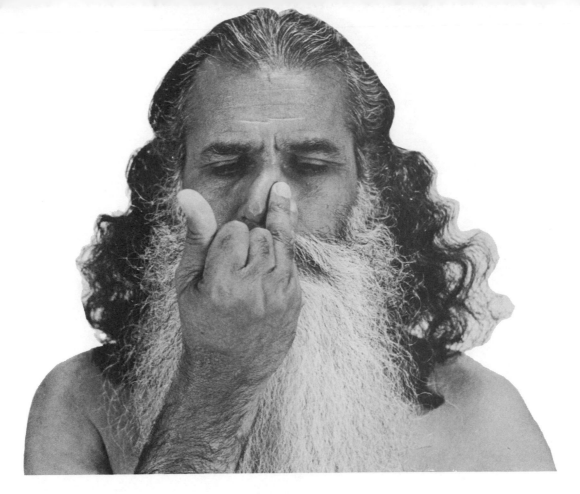

NĀDI SUDDHI—*Left Side*

you to start a new round. Please note that there is no retention, nor any fixed time for the inhalation or exhalation in Stage I of the practice.

Practice this for a few weeks and get used to it.

Stage II: You may now start measuring the time of your Puraka and Rechaka. At the beginning, make sure that the Rechaka takes a longer time than the Puraka, slowly creating a ratio of 1:2 between the Puraka and Rechaka. For example, if you inhale for a count of five, exhale for a count of ten. The speed of the outgoing air is half the speed of the incoming air. Practice the 5:10 ratio for a week and increase it, week by week, to 6:12, 7:14, etc., until you reach 10:20.

In measuring the time of the Puraka and Rechaka, count "Om 1, Om 2, Om 3, etc.," mentally, instead of simply "1, 2, 3, etc.," as this will be very beneficial as well as give you the exact number of seconds.

After reaching the 10:20 ratio, do not increase the duration of the Puraka and Rechaka. Instead, maintain this ratio, and increase the number of breaths to from thirty to fifty times. Once you come to this final stage of Nādi Suddhi, you will really enjoy its benefits.

BENEFITS: Nādi Suddhi brings lightness of body, alertness of the mind, good appetite, proper digestion, and sound sleep.

NOTE: Only at the final stage of this exercise are you fit to go into further types of pranāyāmā that include retention (Kumbaka). If you ignore this and proceed to practice the other breathing exercises in a hurry, no Yoga teacher could stop you from falling into danger.

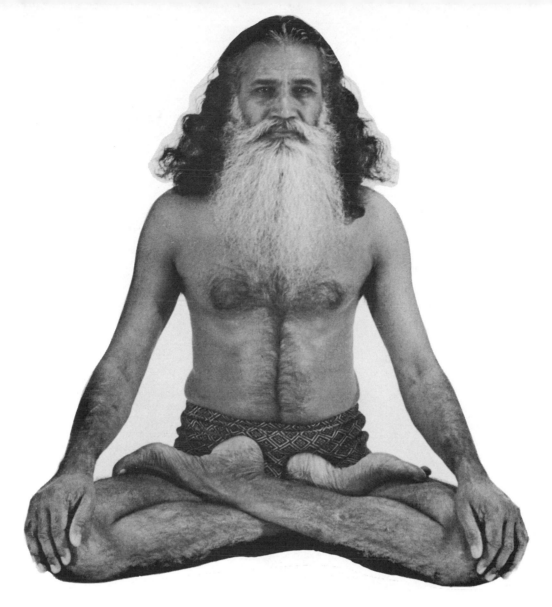

KAPĀLABHĀTI

3 / KAPĀLABHĀTI OR THE SKULL SHINING

TECHNIQUE: Do rapid Rechaka and Puraka, alternating the two forcefully as many times as you can comfortably do, giving equal force to both the exhalation and the inhalation. There is no retention. Kapālabhāti could be treated as preliminary to Bastrika (bellows breathing).

CAUTION: Do not hurry this breathing at any point. If dizziness results, stop the practice.

TIME: Do three rounds. Start with a few expulsions to one round, gradually increasing the number according to your capacity.

NOTE: Kapālabhāti is so called because it cleanses the nādis in the skull.

Although Kapālabhāti is considered a Kriya or cleansing practice, it is part of the prānāyāma section as it is helpful in learning Bastrika.

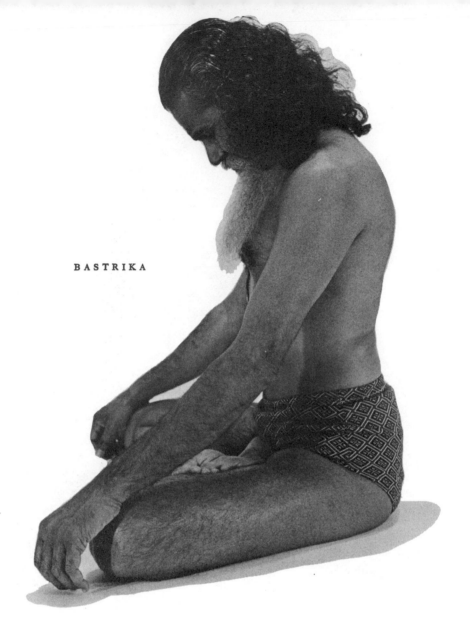

BASTRIKA

4 / BASTRIKA OR THE BELLOWS BREATHING

TECHNIQUE: Do rapid Rechaka and Puraka as in Kapālabhāti, as many times as you can comfortably do, but give slightly extra force to Rechaka. When you have finished, exhale completely and inhale slowly, filling the lungs. Hold the breath. While the breath is being held, bend the neck, bringing the chin as close to the chest as possible. Retain the breath as long as you comfortably can. Then raise the head up slowly and exhale the breath evenly through the nose. This constitutes one round of Bastrika.

CAUTION: Do not hurry this breathing at any point, nor retain the breath beyond your capacity. If dizziness results, stop the practice.

TIME: Start with a few expulsions to one round, gradually increasing the number according to your capacity, up to three rounds.

BENEFITS: Bastrika brings heat to the body when it is cold. It improves digestion, removes phlegm, and helps in curing asthma and consumption. It exhilarates the blood circulation and stimulates the entire body quickly.

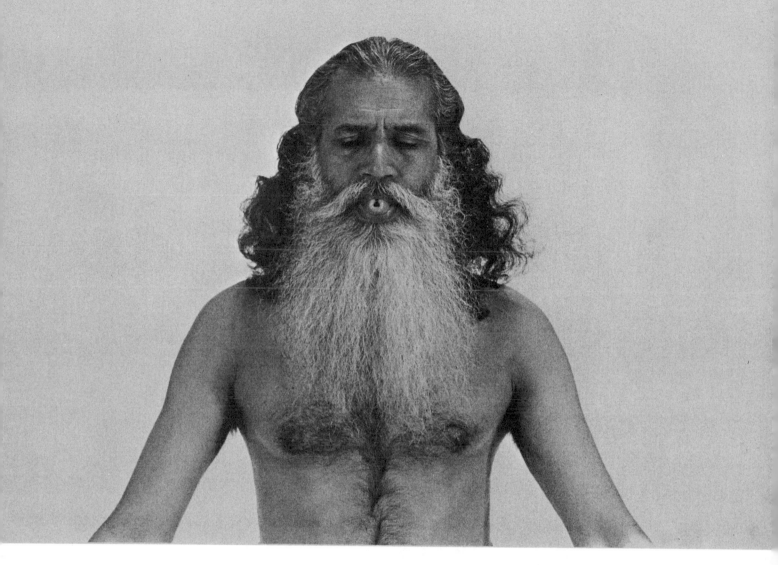

SITALI

5 / SITALI OR THE COOLING BREATH

TECHNIQUE: Fold the tongue lengthwise like a tube. Project the tip of the tongue outside of the mouth. Draw the air in through this tube with a hissing sound. Fill the lungs to capacity. Draw the tongue in, close the mouth and retain the air as long as is comfortably possible. Exhale slowly through the nose. This constitutes one round.

TIME: Do up to three rounds.

BENEFITS: Sitali is a very easy device for cooling off the body. It helps to remove heat, thirst, hunger, and sleep.

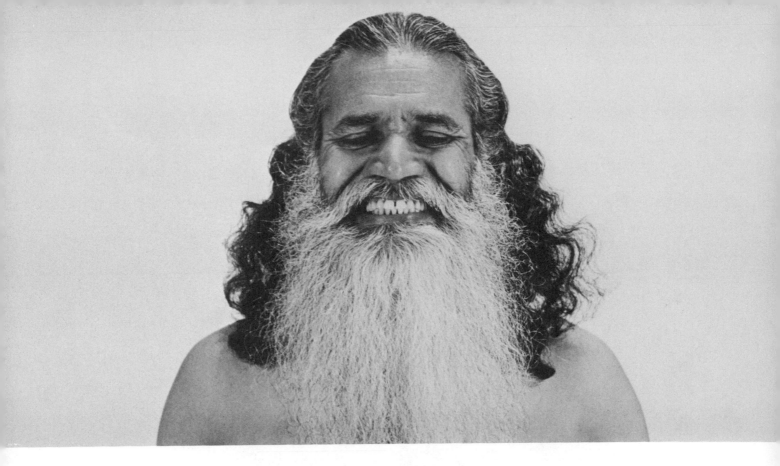

SITKĀRI

6 / SITKĀRI OR THE WHEEZING BREATH

TECHNIQUE: Fold the tongue back (upward), breadthwise around the middle so that the tip of the tongue touches the upper palate. Clench the teeth. Suck in the breath through the clenched teeth with a hissing sound. Fill the lungs to capacity. This constitutes one round.
TIME: Do up to three rounds.
BENEFITS: The same as for Sitali, as well as strengthening of the gums.

7 / BRAHMARI OR THE HUMMING BEE

TECHNIQUE: Inhale through both nostrils, filling the lungs to capacity. Exhale, humming with the sound of a bee. Produce this sound within the head, feeling it on or behind the soft palate. Repeat as many times as possible. When performing Brahmari, inhale deeply and exhale with the humming.

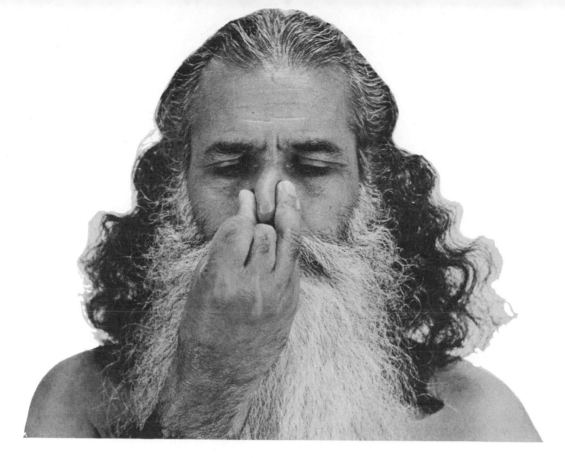

SUKHA PURVAKA

8 / SUKHA PURVAKA OR THE EASY, COMFORTABLE BREATH

TECHNIQUE:

Stage I: The technique of Sukha Purvaka is quite easy once you are acquainted with Nādi Suddhi—the only difference between the two being the Kumbaka, or retention of breath, after each Puraka, during the former practice.

Start with as short a duration of Kumbaka as possible, say a proportion of 10:10:20 between Puraka, Kumbaka, and Rechaka. With this ratio, do five or six breathings and gradually week by week, add three or four, until the number of prānāyāmās is between thirty and fifty a day in two or three sittings.

Stage II: Increase the ratio to 10:15:20. Again, start with five or six breathings, gradually working up to from thirty to fifty a day. After you have reached from thirty to fifty breathings a day, increase the Kumbaka gradually by five counts at a time.

Stage III: The final stage would be a ratio of 10:40:20. This should be reached very slowly, bit by bit, over a period of from nine to twelve months. After this is reached, you need not alter the ratio, but increase the number of prānāyāmās to as many as you like.

While performing Sukha Purvaka, feel that all the divine qualities, such as peace, joy, love, and mercy, are entering your system along with the breath. Likewise, feel that all the devilish qualities of greed, lust, anger, and jealousy are being driven out along with the exhalation. Such mental suggestions are of great benefit to the practitioner.

BENEFITS: Sukha Purvaka has all the benefits of Nādi Suddhi plus it enriches the quality of the blood and ensures perfect physical health. The mind becomes very clear and steady, enabling good concentration.

9 / UJJAYI OR THE HISSING BREATH

TECHNIQUE: Sit in a meditative pose, preferably Padmāsana (lotus pose) or a comparably accomplished pose. Close the mouth. After a complete exhalation, inhale slowly and evenly while partially closing the glottis, located at the base of the nasal passage, so that a continuous, soft hissing sound is heard within the head. This sound should be of even pitch and intensity throughout. Avoid all friction in the nose. Inhale, expanding the lungs to capacity. Retain as long as is comfortably possible. Then, block the right nostril with the hand and slowly exhale through the left nostril. When done while standing or walking, exhalation can be done through both nostrils.

CAUTION: Do not breathe hurriedly or in jerks. The breathing should be done evenly throughout. Even the least strain is to be avoided.

TIME: There is no time restriction. One can practice this at any time and for as long as one wishes.

BENEFITS: Ujjayi relieves heat in the head and increases digestive fire. It helps in the cure of asthma, consumption, and other pulmonary diseases. It adds luster to the face.

NOTE: Ancient authorities on Yoga claim that by its practice death and decay can be overcome.

"Prānāyāma is a scientific remedy against the evil tendency of the mind and the sense organs."

—MANU SMRUTHI (VI 71, 72)

PART SIX

BANDHAS

"Bandha" means "binding" or "lock." Practicing the bandhas binds the prana, or vital energy, and directs it toward the different nerve centers and glands, according to the concentration.

Bandhas should be learned under personal guidance and practiced with great care.

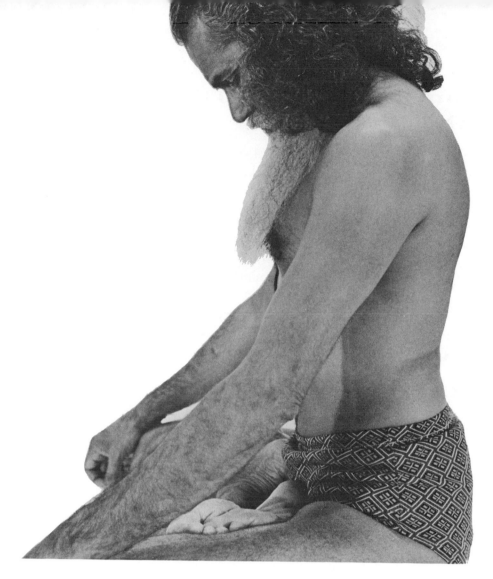

JĀLANDHRA BANDHA

1 / JĀLANDHRA BANDHA OR THE CHIN LOCK

TECHNIQUE: Bend the head and neck so that the chin presses against the chest, creating the chin lock. This is practiced during prānāyāma, whenever the Kumbaka (retention of breath) is done.

BENEFITS: Jālandhra Bandha makes holding the breath during prānāyāma easy. It also helps in increasing the pressure of the breath during prānāyāma.

2 / MOOLA BANDHA OR THE ANUS LOCK

TECHNIQUE: Contract the sphincters, situated at the rectum. Feel as if you are sucking the entire rectum upward, and hold it. This bandha can be practiced during prāṇāyāma.

CAUTION: When this lock is practiced, the genitals, too, are drawn inward. Care must be taken, therefore, not to strain too much.

BENEFITS: Moola Bandha directs the sex energy upward, from its normal downward course. It helps to keep in check nocturnal emissions and aids in maintaining celibacy. It also increases the benefit of prāṇāyāma during retention.

3 / UDDHIYĀNA BANDHA OR THE STOMACH LIFT

Please see Cultural Poses, Section I, page 76.

4 / BANDHA TRAYA OR THE TRIPLE LOCK

TECHNIQUE: Bandha Traya is a combination of Jālandhra Bandha (chin lock), Moola Bandha (anus lock), and Uddhiyāna Bandha (stomach lift), and is practiced during prāṇāyāma. When inhaling and retaining the breath, practice Moola Bandha. When retaining, practice Jālandhra Bandha, along with Moola Bandha; and, during exhalation, practice Uddhiyāna.

CAUTION: As Bandha Traya is a powerful and strenuous practice, it should be learned properly with the help of an adept, and only after the practitioner has perfected Nādi Suddhi and other prāṇāyāmās. Great care must be taken so that there is no undue exertion.

BENEFITS: Bandha Traya charges the whole body with prana. It helps in unifying the prana and the apana (the upward and downward movements of the vital energy). It also acts as an aid in awakening the psychic force, Kundalini.

[154]

PART SEVEN

MUDRAS

"Mudra" means "seal," and the mudras are concerned with the mind. Practicing the mudras keeps the mind fixed on the points over which they are applied.

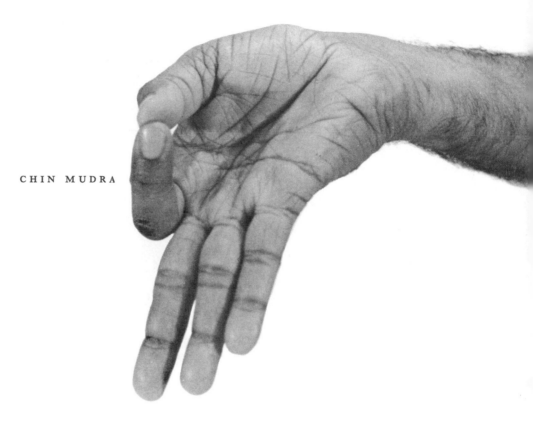

CHIN MUDRA

1 / CHIN MUDRA OR THE SYMBOL OF WISDOM

TECHNIQUE: Rest the hands on the corresponding knees. Stretch out the upturned palms. On each hand, touch the tip of the thumb with the tip of the index finger. Point the remaining three fingers on each hand downward.

This mudra can be practiced only when the hands are not being used (as occurs in closing the nostrils during Nādi Suddhi, or in counting the number of prānāyāmās done).

BENEFITS: Chin Mudra helps in reminding the practitioner of the purpose of life, during meditation. It can also bring added benefit to the practice of prānāyāma.

NOTE: You may wonder why the name "Symbol of Wisdom" has been given to this mudra. It is because all the fingers of the hand represent something. The thumb represents the higher or Universal Self. The index finger represents the individual self; the middle finger, the ego; the third or ring finger, the illusion of the mind; and the fourth or pinky, the worldly actions and their reactions. During Chin Mudra, the individual self renounces all worldliness and rises up toward the higher Self. While watching the efforts of the individual self, the higher Self gracefully bends down to meet it. So, the union of the Universal and individual selves is symbolized by this mudra, the Symbol of Wisdom.

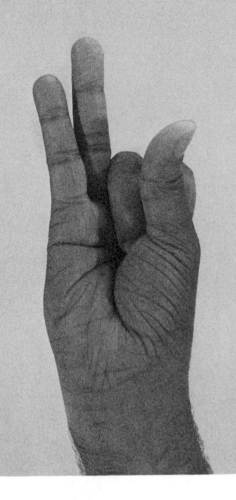

VISHNU MUDRA

2 / VISHNU MUDRA OR THE SEAL OF VISHNU

TECHNIQUE: Close the fingers and look at the right palm. Hold down the index and middle fingers with the root of the thumb. Raise the other two fingers.

Vishnu Mudra is used during prānāyāma when the nostrils are changed or closed, as in Nādi Suddhi. In this particular case, the thumb is used to close the right nostril and the last two fingers are used to close the left nostril.

BENEFITS: This mudra makes the changing of the right and left nostrils, and closing them, easy during prānāyāma.

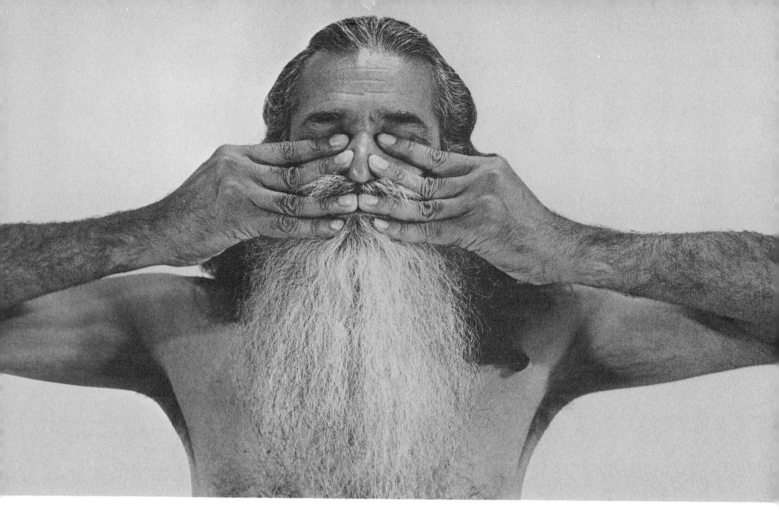

SHANMUKHI MUDRA

3 / SHANMUKHI MUDRA OR THE SIX-WAY SEAL

TECHNIQUE: Sit in any one of the meditative poses and raise the elbows sideways to shoulder level. Close the ears with the thumbs, the eyes with the index fingers, by placing the fingers near the lower eyelid. Adjust the middle fingers on either side of the nostrils, ready to close one or both, when necessary. Close the mouth by pressing the upper lip with the ring fingers and the lower with the pinkies. Then, take a slow, deep inhalation. Hold the breath and close the nostrils with the middle fingers. At the same time, perform Moola Bandha (anus lock), thereby shutting the anus and genital opening.

Retain this mudra as long as you easily can. Release the Moola Bandha and the nostrils and exhale slowly.

CAUTION: Great care should be taken during the entire process to make sure that the eyelids are not pressed too hard, or that the Moola Bandha is done beyond your capacity. As this is a very advanced practice, one should not attempt it before mastering the standard Yoga postures and Nādi Suddhi prānāyāma.

BENEFITS: Shanmukhi Mudra is a great aid toward the practice of pratyahara, or sense control, as the mind is introverted to help concentration.

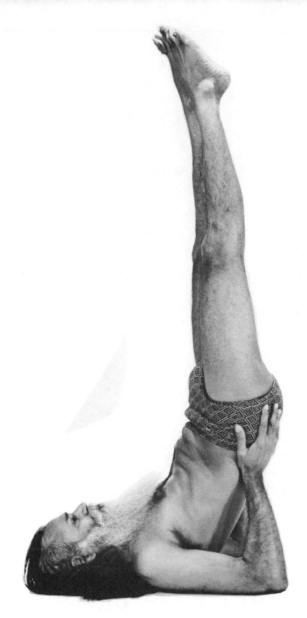

VIPAREETHAKARANI MUDRA

4 / VIPAREETHAKARANI MUDRA
OR THE REVERSING SEAL

TECHNIQUE: Lie on the back, with the hands alongside the body. Slowly raise the legs off the floor and then the hips. Raise the forearms to support the back with the hands, slightly above the buttocks.

CAUTION: You need not support the trunk of the body, as in Sarvāgāsana (shoulder stand). Let it be at a straight angle.

BENEFITS: This mudra increases the digestive fire and renews youthful vitality.

NOTE: The sun, in the human body, is situated below at the navel's root, and the moon is situated up at the roof of the palate. By this mudra, the sun takes the upper place, and the moon the lower. Thus the name "Reversing Seal."

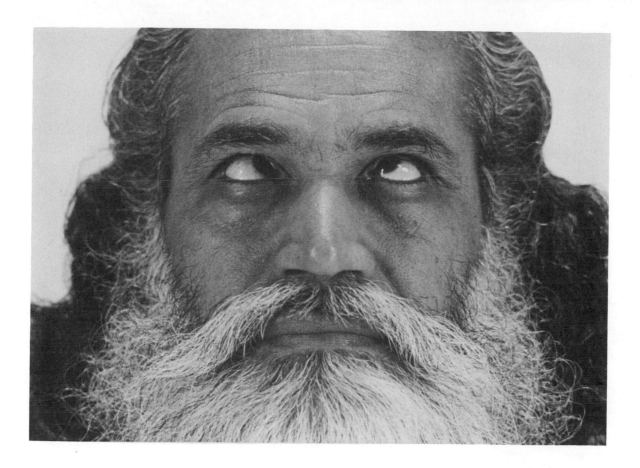

SĀMBAVI MUDRA

5 / SĀMBAVI MUDRA, BRUMADHYA DRISHTI, OR THE GAZE BETWEEN THE EYEBROWS

TECHNIQUE: Become aware of the Ajna Chakra, the space between the eyebrows. Bring to this spot a mental picture of your Ishtha Devatha, Beloved Deity. The physical eyes may be half-opened and may gently blink.

Another way of doing Sāmbavi Mudra is to gently direct the vision upward and inward, gazing on the space between the eyebrows. Feel that you are in contact with your Ishtha Devatha and meditate upon him or it.

CAUTION: The first technique is safer than the second. Be careful not to strain the eyes. After the practice, close them until they are well rested.

BENEFITS: This mudra helps to keep the mind one-pointed. It is said that it also aids the cure of insomnia.

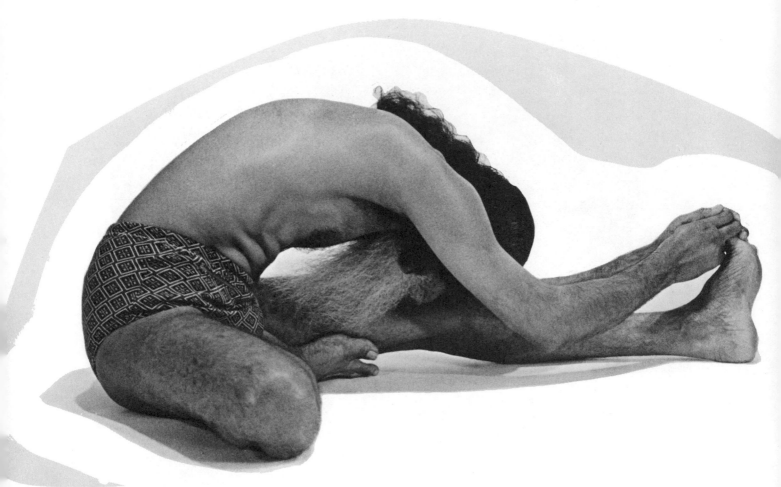

MAHĀ MUDRA

6 / MAHĀ MUDRA OR THE GREAT SEAL

TECHNIQUE: Sit on the floor, with the legs stretched forward. Bend the left leg, bringing the heel under the anus. Feel the pressure on the anus. Bend forward, catching the right toe with the hands. Inhale and retain the breath, practicing Jālandhra Bandha (chin lock). Fix the gaze between the eyebrows. Bend forward more, without any strain, to your maximum limit. Hold the position as long as you can comfortably do so. Release the pose and the breath. Repeat the pose, bending the right leg.

BENEFITS: Mahā Mudra aids the cure of consumption, hemorrhoids or piles, enlargement of the spleen, constipation, indigestion, and various abdominal disorders.

NOTE: The posture in this mudra is almost the same as Jānushirshāsana (head-to-knee pose), but without the retention of the breath.

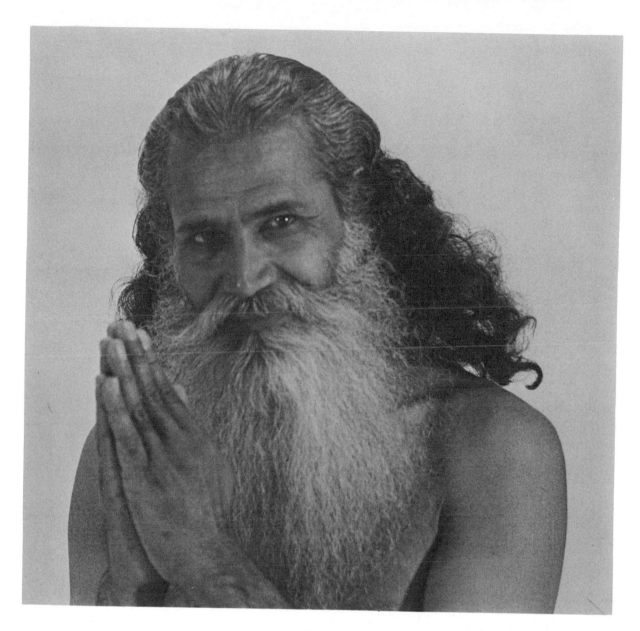

NAMASKĀRA MUDRA

7 / NAMASKĀRA MUDRA OR THE SALUTATION SEAL

TECHNIQUE: Bring the palms together so that they touch each other opposite the middle of the chest, with the fingers pointing upward.

NOTE: This hand position is the traditional Hindu way of greeting and saluting.

8 / ASWINI MUDRA OR THE HORSE SEAL

TECHNIQUE: Contract the anal sphincters, situated at the rectum. Feel as if you are sucking the entire rectum up, and hold it. Then, contract and dilate the sphincters a number of times.

Aswini Mudra may be practiced in any meditative pose, or in Sarvāngāsana (shoulder stand) or Sirshāsana (head stand).

BENEFITS: This mudra helps to get rid of constipation and piles. It tones up the seminal glands and the nerves of that area.

NOTE: Aswini Mudra and Moola Bandha are the same, except during the latter there is no alternate contraction and dilation.

9 / YOGA MUDRA OR THE YOGIC SEAL

Please see Cultural Poses, Section I, page 82.

"*Do not mistake laziness for relaxation. The lazy man is inactive. He has no inclination for work. He is full of lethargy and inertia. He is dull. Whereas a man who practices relaxation takes only rest. He has vigor, strength, vitality, and endurance. He never allows even a small amount of energy to trickle away. He accomplishes wonderful work gracefully in a minimum amount of time.*"

—SWAMI SIVANANDA

PART EIGHT

SHAT KRIYAS
or
THE SIX PURIFICATORY EXERCISES

The definition of "Kriya" is "action." In Hatha Yoga, kriya specifically means a purificatory technique. The definition of "Shat" is "six." These six techniques given, when practiced properly, help in maintaining perfect physical health. It is a subjective approach to clean the system of impurities.

I | DHAUTI OR STOMACH CLEANSING

There are four types of Dhauti:
1. Vastra or Cloth Dhauti
2. Jala or Water Dhauti
3. Agnisāra or Fire Dhauti
4. Vārisāra or Wind Dhauti

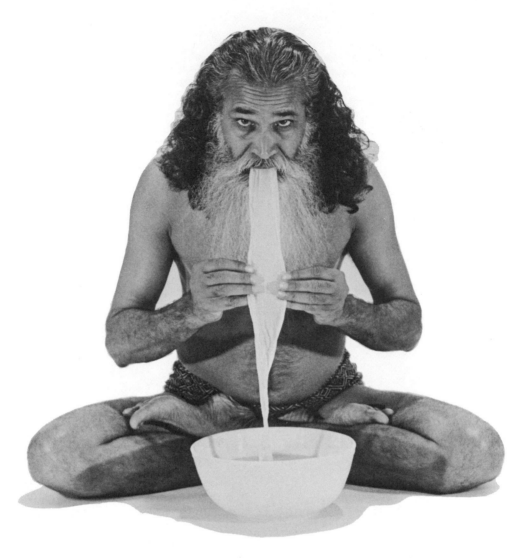

VASTRA DHAUTI

1 / VASTRA OR CLOTH DHAUTI

TECHNIQUE: Take a clean, fine piece of cloth—three inches wide by fifteen feet long. The edges should be sewn, and there should be no loose threads. It should be washed in soap and water. For your practice, dip it into tepid water and squeeze it out. Then, slowly take one end of it into your mouth and swallow just one foot's length. Let it stay there for a few minutes. Slowly, draw it out. Do not be rough or in a hurry. Gradually increase the length until you can swallow all fifteen feet.

CAUTION: Make sure to do this on an empty stomach.

BENEFITS: Vastra Dhauti aids flabby phlegmatic conditions. It helps to cure bile, phlegm, and gastritis and other gastric disorders.

[168]

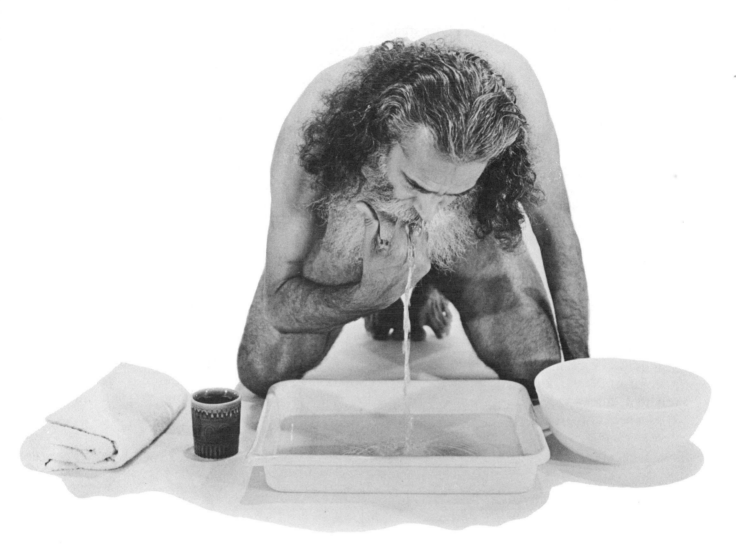

JALA DHAUTI

2 / JALA OR WATER DHAUTI

TECHNIQUE: Drink four or five glasses of lukewarm water, preferably with a little salt in it. After a few minutes, do rigorous Uddhiyāna Bandha (stomach lift). Shake the intestines well. Press the stomach with the hand and then vomit out the water. If the water will not come out naturally, use the fingers to get it out.

BENEFITS: All impurities, phlegm, and bile will be washed out.

3 / AGNISĀRA OR FIRE DHAUTI

TECHNIQUE: Either sit or stand. Using a little force, exhale fully. Holding the breath out, pump the abdominal muscles in and out in quick succession, as many times as can be comfortably done. Gradually increase the number of strokes, even up to one hundred times if you can comfortably do so. Stop pumping before becoming exhausted, and allow the breath to go in. This process makes one round.

CAUTION: The stomach lift should not be held beyond one's capacity. Agnisāra Dhauti is to be avoided in cases of circulatory disturbances and serious abdominal troubles.

TIME: Agnisāra Dhauti can be practiced for two or three rounds at a time.

BENEFITS: This pose increases the digestive power and helps to cure all types of gastric complaints. It increases peristalsis of the bowels and helps to cure constipation. It also aids in reducing fat in the belly.

NOTE: This is called Agnisāra Dhauti, or fire cleansing, because it increases the gastric fire.

4 / VĀRISĀRA OR WIND DHAUTI

TECHNIQUE: Either sit or stand. Stretch the neck forward, relaxing the throat muscles. Suck air into the mouth and swallow it. Fill up the stomach as much as can comfortably be done. Practice Nauli Kriya (isolation and rolling of the abdominal recti) and Uddhiyāna Bandha (stomach lift). After a while, belch the air out. If some air escapes through the anus, let it go.

BENEFITS: Helps in clearing out gas from the stomach.

II | BASTI OR COLON CLEANSING

There are two types of Basti:
1. Sthala or Ground Basti
2. Jala or Water Basti

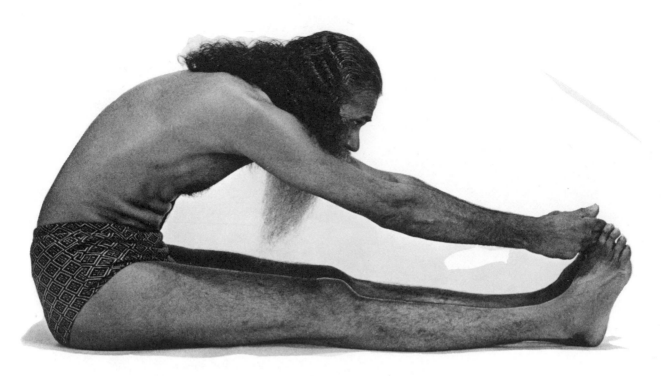

STHALA BASTI

1 / STHALA OR GROUND BASTI

TECHNIQUE: Sit on the floor, with the legs stretched out. Hold the toes with the corresponding hands. Bring the head toward the knees as in Paschimothānāsana (forward bend), but do not bend very much. Relax the abdominal muscles and churn them with upward and downward movements. During these movements, if possible, do Moola Bandha (anus lock) contractions.

CAUTION: Sthala Basti should be practiced with an empty stomach. Do not exert yourself when practicing it.

BENEFITS: Sthala Basti helps in relieving gas and in having a free movement of the bowels.

2 / JALA OR WATER BASTI

TECHNIQUE: Squat in a bathtub or in a river, with the water up to the knees. Do Uddhiyāna Bandha (stomach lift) and expel the air from inside the body. Then do Nauli Kriya (isolation and rolling of the abdominal recti). Open the anus by doing Aswini Mudra (horse seal). A vacuum will then be created in the abdomen, and water will immediately be drawn up into the colon. Stand up and expel the indrawn water by doing Uddhiyāna Bandha and Aswini Mudra.

BENEFITS: Jala Basti will clear out accumulations in the intestines.

NOTE: This is more effective than Sthala or Ground Basti. This is only for occasional practice. If you find it difficult to expand the anus and keep it open, insert a well-lubricated, thin plastic or rubber tube of about five inches long into this opening.

III | NETI OR NASAL CLEANSING

There are two types of Neti:
1. Jala or Water Neti
2. Sootra or String Neti

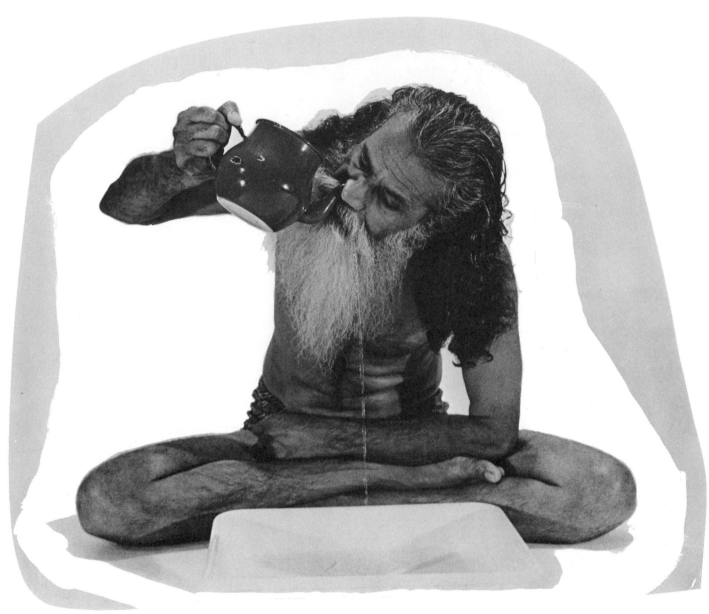

JALA NETI

1 / JALA OR WATER NETI

TECHNIQUE: Draw water in through the nose and spit it out through the mouth. Then, draw water through the mouth and blow out through the nostrils.
BENEFITS: Jala Neti helps prevent colds and cleanses the nasal passages.

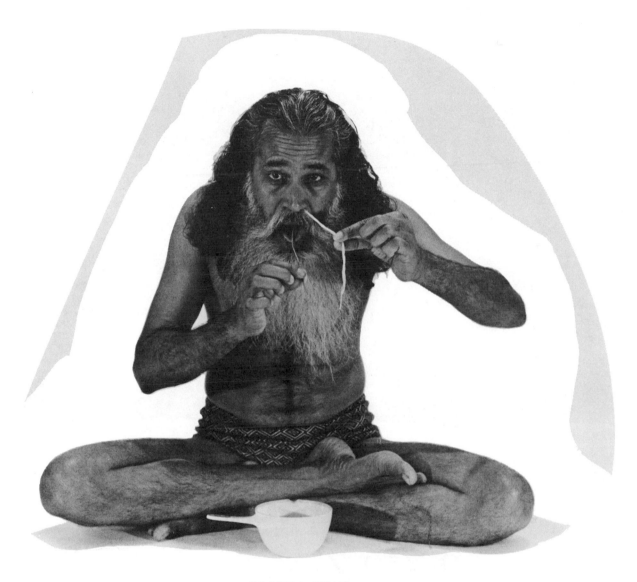

SOOTRA NETI

2 / SOOTRA OR STRING NETI

TECHNIQUE: Take a string, waxed at one end. Insert the waxed end into a nostril, holding the other end in the hand. Inhale slowly and deeply and draw the thread inside. Slowly pull it out. Do this through both nostrils, cleaning them thoroughly.

BENEFITS: This purifies the nostrils so that breathing will be uniform, even, and easy.

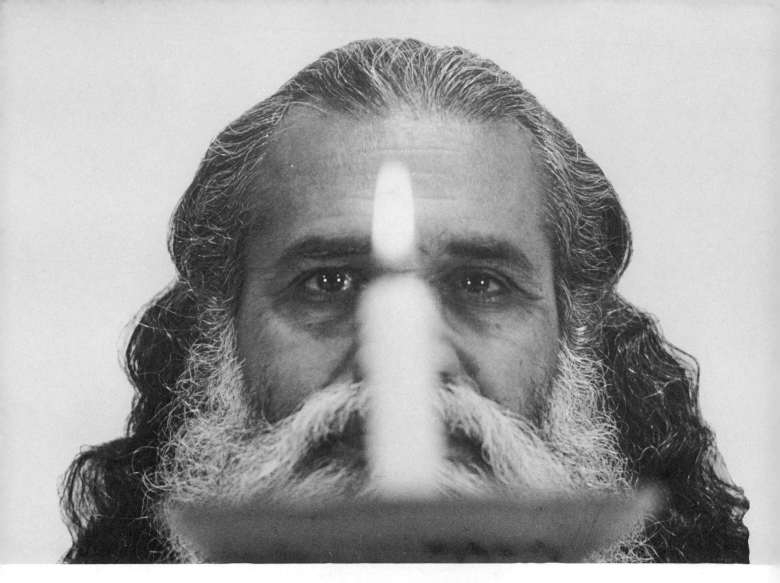

THRATAKAM

IV | THRATAKAM OR GAZING

TECHNIQUE: Thratakam can be done on either external objects or on parts of one's own body. Select a picture of your Beloved Deity, spiritual teacher, or any holy person you choose. You can even select a candle flame, small electric light—any small, bright object, even a dot. Place the object at eye level, neither too far nor too near the eyes, and look at it steadily without blinking for as long as you comfortably can.

When doing Thratakam on parts of the body, normally the tip of the nose or the space between the eyebrows is chosen. These are called Nāsāgra Drishti and Brumadhya Drishti, respectively.

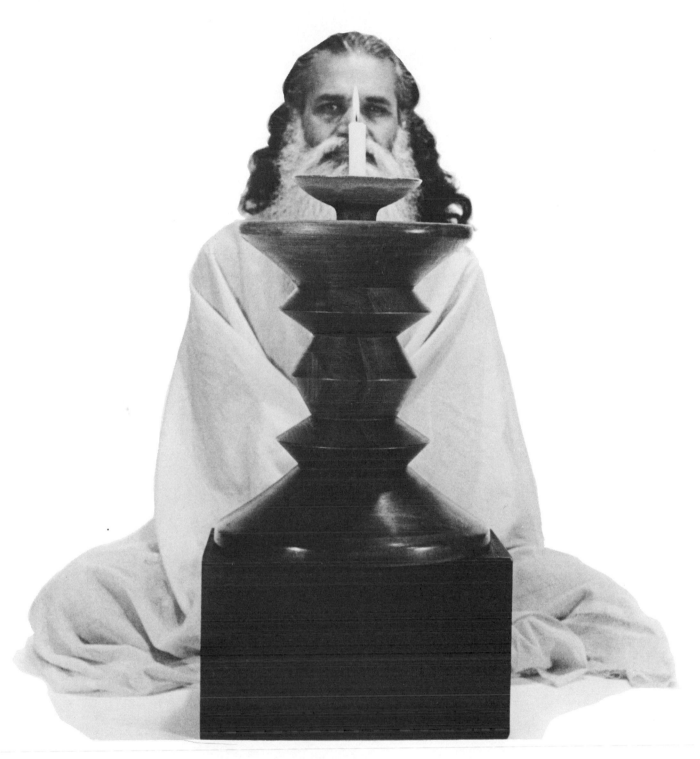

THRATAKAM

CAUTION: Avoid any undue strain to the eyes. Thratakam should be practiced slowly and cautiously. Those persons with eye trouble should consult a Yoga adept before starting this practice.

BENEFITS: This practice develops concentration and helps improve the eyesight.

V | NAULI KRIYA OR THE ISOLATION AND ROLLING OF THE ABDOMINAL RECTI

Please see Cultural Poses, Section I, page 78.

VI | KAPĀLABHĀTI OR THE SKULL SHINING

Please see Prānāyāma, page 145.

APPENDIX

COURSES
FOR
FURTHER
STUDY

Listed below are three suggested courses of practice: Beginner, Intermediate, and Advanced.

First 3 months—Beginner. Repeat each āsana between three and six times, holding each ten seconds per time, with the exceptions noted under Sarvāngāsana, Matsyāsana, Arddha Matsyendrāsana, Arddha Chandrāsana, and Yoga Mudra.

3–6 months—Beginner. Repeat each āsana two to three times, holding each fifteen to twenty seconds per time, with above exceptions.

6 months–1 year—Intermediate. Repeat each āsana once or twice, holding each thirty seconds to one minute per time, with exceptions.

1 year or more—Advanced. Hold all āsanas at least one minute without strain, with noted exceptions.

Poses with asterisks* are to be done daily. All others are optional and may be done to your taste and convenience.

BEGINNER	INTERMEDIATE	ADVANCED
*Nethra Vyāyāmam, Sections I & II (eye exercises)	*Nethra Vyāyāmam, Sections I & II	*Nethra Vyāyāmam, Sections I & II
*Soorya Namaskāram (salutation to the sun)	*Soorya Namaskāram, with dip	*Soorya Namaskāram, with dip

(Of the following Meditative Poses, choose one—Padmasāna, Vajrāsana, Siddhāsana, or Swastikāsana.)

Meditative Poses

*Arddha Padmāsana (half lotus pose)	*Padmāsana (lotus pose)	*Padmāsana
*Vajrāsana (pelvic pose)	*Vajrāsana	*Vajrāsana
*Swastikāsana (favorable pose)	*Swastikāsana	*Swastikāsana
	*Siddhāsana (accomplished pose)	*Siddhāsana
Yoga Battāsana (Yogic belt pose)		

BEGINNER	INTERMEDIATE	ADVANCED
Cultural Poses, Section I		
*Bhujangāsana (cobra pose)	*Bhujangāsana	*Bhujangāsana
*Arddha Salabāsana (half-locust pose)		
*Salabāsana (locust pose)	*Salabāsana	*Salabāsana
*Dhanurāsana (bow pose)	*Dhanurāsana	*Dhanurāsana
*Jānusirshāsana (head-to-knee pose)	*Jānusirshāsana	*Jānusirshāsana
*Paschimothānāsana (forward-bending pose)	*Paschimothānāsana	*Paschimothānāsana
	*Halāsana (plow pose)	*Halāsana
*Sarvāngāsana (shoulder stand)	*Sarvāngāsana	*Sarvāngāsana
		*Padma Sarvāngāsana (lotus shoulder stand)
*Matsyāsana (fish pose)	*Matsyāsana in Padmāsana	*Matsyāsana in Padmāsana
Pavanamuktāsana (wind-eliminating pose)	Pavanamuktāsana	Pavanamuktāsana
*Mayurāsana, Stage I (peacock pose)	*Mayurāsana	*Mayurāsana
		Padma Mayurāsana (lotus peacock pose)
*Arddha Matsyendrāsana (half spinal twist)	*Arddha Matsyendrāsana	*Arddha Matsyendrāsana
Trikonāsana (triangular pose)	Trikonāsana Variation	Trikonāsana Variation
Padahasthāsana (hand-to-feet pose)	Padahasthāsana	Padahasthāsana
	Arddha Chandrāsana (crescent pose)	Arddha Chandrāsana
*Sirshāsana, I–III (head stand)	*Sirshāsana	*Sirshāsana
		Oordhwa Padmāsana (upward lotus pose)
*Uddhiyāna Bandha (stomach lift)	*Uddhiyāna Bandha	*Uddhiyāna Bandha

BEGINNER	INTERMEDIATE	ADVANCED
Cultural Poses, Section I		
*Nauli Kriya (abdominal rolling)	*Nauli Kriya	*Nauli Kriya
*Yoga Mudra (Yogic seal)	*Yoga Mudra	*Yoga Mudra
*Savāsana (corpse pose)	*Savāsana	*Savāsana
Cultural Poses, Section II		
		Ākarshna Dhanurāsana (shooting-bow pose)
	Āñjaneyāsana (monkey pose)	Āñjaneyāsana
	Baddha Jānushirshāsana (bound head-to-knee pose)	Baddha Jānushirshāsana
		Baddha Padmāsana (bound lotus pose)
		Baddha Yoga Mudra (bound Yogic seal)
Badrāsana (gentle pose)	Badrāsana	Badrāsana
		Durvāsāsana (Durvasa's pose)
		Eka Pāda Trikonāsana (single-leg triangle pose)
		Ekapādhasirshāsana (leg-to-head pose)
	Garudāsana (eagle pose)	Garudāsana
		Gharbāsana (child-in-womb pose)
	Gomukhāsana (cow-face pose)	Gomukhāsana
Kakāsana (crow pose)	Kakāsana	Kakāsana
	Karnapeetāsana (ear-to-knee pose)	Karnapeetāsana
		Koormāsana (tortoise pose)
		Kukkutāsana (cock pose)

BEGINNER	INTERMEDIATE	ADVANCED
Cultural Poses, Section II		
Natarājāsana (king dancer pose)	Natarājāsana	Natarājāsana
	Nirālamba Sarvāngāsana (unsupported shoulder stand)	Nirālamba Sarvāngāsana
		Omkārāsana (om pose)
		Padhāngushtāsana (tiptoes pose)
		Parvathāsana (mountain pose)
	Paschima Nāuāsana (forward boat pose)	Paschima Nāuāsana
		Poorna Matsyāsana (full fish pose)
		Poorna Matsyendrāsana (full spinal twist)
		Poorna Supta Vajrāsana (full bent pelvic pose)
		Poorna Utthitha Padmāsana (fully elevated lotus pose)
Poorva Nāuāsana (backward boat pose)	Poorva Nāuāsana	Poorva Nāuāsana
	Sankatāsana (chair pose)	Sankatāsana
	Sasangāsana (rabbit pose)	Sasangāsana
		Sethu Bandhāsana (bridge pose)
	Sethu Bandha Sarvāngāsana (bridge shoulder stand)	Sethu Bandha Sarvāngāsana
Simhāsana (lion pose)	Simhāsana	Simhāsana
	Supta Vajrāsana (bent pelvic pose)	Supta Vajrāsana
	Tolangulāsana (scale pose)	Tolangulāsana

BEGINNER	INTERMEDIATE	ADVANCED
Cultural Poses, Section II		
	Utthitha Dhanurāsana (raised-bow pose)	Utthitha Dhanurāsana Utthitha Koormāsana (lifted tortoise pose)
	Utthitha Padmāsana (lifted lotus pose)	Utthitha Padmāsana
		Utthitha Paschimothānāsana (lifted forward-bending pose)
Vajrāsana (pelvic pose)	Vajrāsana	Vajrāsana
		Vajra Tolangulāsana (pelvic scale pose)
		Vakrāsana (crooked pose)
	Vāthayānāsana (foot-and-knee pose)	Vāthayānāsana
Vrikshāsana (tree pose)	Vrikshāsana	Vrikshāsana
		Yoga Nidrāsana (Yogic sleep)
Pranāyāmās		
Deergha Sirvasam (deep breathing)		
*Nādi Suddhi (nerve purification)		
*Kapālabhāti (skull shining)		
	*Bastrika (bellows breathing)	*Bastrika
Sitali (cooling breath)	Sitali	Sitali
Sitkāri (wheezing breath)	Sitkāri	Sitkāri
Brahmari (humming bce)	Brahmari	Brahmari
	*Sukha Purvaka (easy, comfortable breath)	*Sukha Purvaka
	*Ujjayi (hissing breath)	*Ujjayi

BEGINNER	INTERMEDIATE	ADVANCED
Bandhas		
	Jālandhra Bandha (chin lock)	Jālandhra Bandha
		Moola Bandha (anus lock)
		Bandha Traya (triple lock)
Mudras		
Chin Mudra (symbol of wisdom)	Chin Mudra	Chin Mudra
Vishnu Mudra (seal of Vishnu)	Vishnu Mudra	Vishnu Mudra
		Shanmukhi Mudra (six-way seal)
	Vipareethakarani Mudra (reversing seal)	Vipareethakarani Mudra
Sāmbavi Mudra (gaze between the eyebrows)	Sāmbavi Mudra	Sāmbavi Mudra
		Mahā Mudra (great seal)
		Aswini Mudra (horse seal)
Kriyas		
		Vastra Dhauti (cloth cleansing)
	Jala Dhauti (water cleansing)	Jala Dhauti
	Agnisāra Dhauti (fire cleansing)	Agnisāra Dhauti
	Vārisāra Dhauti (wind cleansing)	Vārisāra Dhauti
	Sthala Basti (ground cleansing)	Sthala Basti
	Jala Basti (water cleansing)	Jala Basti
Jala Neti (water cleansing)	Jala Neti	Jala Neti
	Sootra Neti (string cleansing)	Sootra Neti

BEGINNER	INTERMEDIATE	ADVANCED
Thratakam (gazing)	Thratakam	Thratakam

If you wish any further information regarding your Yogic practice, please contact one of the following centers:

Integral Yoga Institutes

New York, N.Y. 10011	227 West 13 St.
New York, N.Y. 10024	500 West End Ave.
Los Angeles, Cal. 90048	6117 Warner Drive
San Francisco, Cal. 94110	770 Dolores St.
Santa Cruz, Cal. 95060	20 Granite Creek Road
Boulder, Colo. 80302	2109 Bluff St.
Washington, D.C. 20008	2445 Porter St. N.W.
Detroit, Mich. 48221	16535 Livernois
Hartford, Conn. 06105	467 Farmington Ave.
Garfield, N.J. 07026	5 Clark St.
Dallas, Texas 75220	9453 Lake North Circle
Montreal, Quebec 108	3551 Jeanne Maue
Brussels, Belgium	286 Chemin de Vleurgat
Paris 6, France	47 Quai des Grands Augustins
Bern, Switzerland 3000	Bubenbergplatz 12
La-Chaux-de-Fonds, Switzerland 2300	11, rue de College
Fribourg, Switzerland 1700	13A, rue Locarno
Lausanne, Switzerland 1012	24, Ch. des Daillettes

Integral Yoga Groups

Columbia, Mo. 65201	215 Ripley Ave.
Carrboro, N.C. 27510	113 Pine St.

Satchidananda Ashrams

Yogaville East	Box 108, Pomfret Center, Conn. 06259
Yogaville West	Star Route, Middletown, Cal. 95461